Zur Geschichte der Hypophysenhormone

Zur Geschichte der Hypophysenhormone

Gerhard Bettendorf

Prof. Dr. med. Gerhard Bettendorf
Friedrich-Kirsten-Straße 19
22391 Hamburg

Die Deutsche Bibliothek – CIP-Einheitsaufnahme

Bettendorf, Gerhard:

Zur Geschichte der Hypophysenhormone / Gerhard Bettendorf.
– Stuttgart : Thieme, 1996
ISBN 3-13-104571-X

© 1996 Georg Thieme Verlag
Rüdigerstraße 14
70469 Stuttgart
Printed in Germany
Satz: DataSatz Roßberg, Metzingen
Druck: Grammlich, Pliezhausen
Buchbinderei: Dollinger, Metzingen
ISBN 3-13-104571-X

Inhalt

Die Publikation wurde durch eine großzügige Unterstützung der Nourypharma, Herrn W. Sassenrath, ermöglicht.
M. Breckwoldt und dem Thieme-Verlag, Herrn Ch. Staehr und Herrn P. Schmidt danke ich für die effiziente Realisierung.

Einleitung

Geschichte schreiben ist immer eine bedenkliche Sache. Denn bei dem redlichsten Vorsatz kommt man in Gefahr unredlich zu sein; ja wer eine solche Darstellung unternimmt erklärt zu Voraus, daß er manches ins Licht, manches in Schatten rücken wird (Goethe im Vorwort zur Farbenlehre).

Der zeitliche Beginn der Erforschung der Hypophyse und ihrer Hormone fällt mit dem Anfang unseres Jahrhunderts zusammen.

Eine zusammenfassende Darstellung der Hypophysen-Hormon-Forschung liegt bisher nicht vor. Ich habe versucht anhand der Originalarbeiten die Entwicklungen im zeitlichen Ablauf von den Anfängen bis heute zusammenzustellen. Von dieser etwa 90jährigen Zeitspanne habe ich fast die Hälfte zunächst beobachtend, später selbst experimentell und klinisch involviert, miterlebt. Grundlage für die vorliegende Zusammenstellung war eine über die Jahre durchgeführte Sammlung der Publikationen und der persönliche Kontakt zu einer großen Zahl der auf diesem Gebiet arbeitenden Wissenschaftler.

Ausführliche Biographien der meisten Forscher auf dem Gebiet der Hypophysenhormone finden sich in dem von mir herausgegebenen Buch „Zur Geschichte der Endokrinologie und Reproduktionsmedizin" (1995).

Auch wenn der Historiker (*Lichtenthaeler*, 1987) feststellt „Medizingeschichte ist viel zu schwer für Mediziner", hoffe ich, daß diese Zusammenstellung interessierte Leser findet, die ein Gespür für die geschichtliche Entwicklung haben.

In seiner Antrittsvorlesung 1963 in Hamburg läßt *Charles Lichtenthaeler* die moderne Medizin mit *Francois Magendie* (1783–1855), dem Lehrer von *Claude Bernard* (1813–1878), beginnen. Seit dieser Zeit „stimmen die historischen Tatsachen, die wir in den Lehrbüchern und anderen Veröffentlichungen gewahren, fast stets mit der Wirklichkeit überein. Die frühere ‚literarische Periode' mit ihrer unentwirrbaren Vermischung von Wahrheit und Irrtum hat somit ein Ende gefunden. Und die Masse der entdeckten Tatsachen ist immer größer geworden, denn man huldigte der Objektivität und auch der Forschung." Die Frage, „Warum Medizingeschichte" beantwortet *Lichtenthaeler* in der ersten Vorlesung in seinem Lehrbuch 1987: „Diese Disziplin ist neben Pathologie, Klinik und Berufskunde ein Fundament des medizinischen Unterrichts. Neben der medizinischen Wissenschaft und der ärztlichen Ethik gibt es eine spezifische ärztliche Bildung, die vor allem durch das Studium der medizinischen Vergangenheit vermittelt wird. Fachliches Wissen allein macht aus Ihnen nur Gesundheitstechniker und -funktionäre; *José Ortega Y Gasset* sprach einst vom ‚spezialisierten Barbaren'. Erst durch das historische Bewußtsein reifen Sie zu wahren ärztlichen Persönlichkeiten heran."

Mit den klassischen Experimenten von *Arnold Adolph Berthold,* Hofrat und Professor für Physiologie in Göttingen von 1849, setzt die Geschichte der Endokrinologie ein. *Berthold* zeigte, daß eine Wirkung von den Hoden auf den Hahnenkamm über das Blut vermittelt wird. Der Begriff „Innere Sekretion" wurde 1855 von *Claude Bernard,* Professor der Physiologie an der Sorbonne, erstmalig verwendet. *Ernest Henry Starling,* Mediziner und Physiologe in London, prägte zusammen mit dem Physiologen *William Bate Hardy* und dem Cambridger Altphilologen *W. T. Vesey* 1905 den Ausdruck „Hormon". *Arthur Biedl,* Pathologe in Wien, gab seinem Buch 1910 den Titel „Innere Sekretion".

Die Entwicklung der Kenntnisse der Hypophysenvorderlappenhormone ist exemplarisch für den Fortgang der endokrinologischen Wissenschaft. Am Anfang stand die anatomische Beschreibung der jeweiligen Drüse, wobei teilweise über deren Funktion spekuliert wurde. Meist folgten klinische und biologische Beobachtungen, die einen Hinweis auf die Bedeutung des Organs für den Organismus ermöglichten und Vermutungen über funktionelle Abläufe entstehen ließen. Die Verbreitung dieser Befunde und deren akademische Diskussion führte dann zu den entscheidenden Experimenten von Physiologen und Klinikern, meist Gynäkologen in einigen wenigen Zentren. Es ist erstaunlich, wie dann in kurzer Zeit von Klinikern versucht wurde, die Resultate der experimentellen Untersuchungen Ende der 20er–30er Jahre für die Medizin nutzbringend einzusetzen. Wissenschaftlich verlangsamte sich der Fortschritt etwa 20 Jahre, bis dann etwa 1950 beginnend wieder ein Schub einsetzte, der mit Unterbrechungen bis heute anhält. Die enthusiasti-

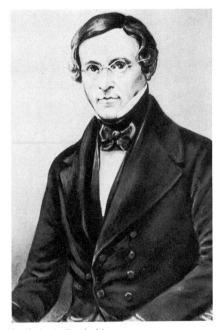

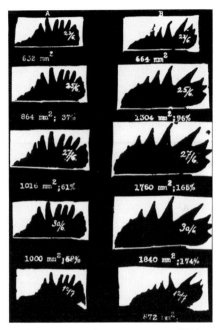

Prof. A. A. Berthold

Größenzunahme des Kammes zeigt Wirksamkeit des eingespritzten Hormons

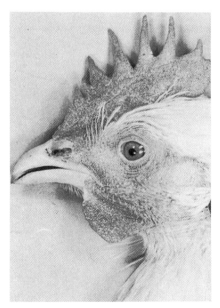

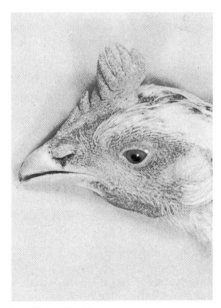

Der Kamm des Hahnes

Der Kamm des Kapauns

A. Berthold (1803–1861): Zoologe, Anatom in Göttingen. Experimenteller Beweis einer inneren Sekretion; 1849: „Transplantation der Hoden".

sche Aufnahme des neuen Wissens zu Anfang ebbte später vorübergehend merklich ab. Die Vermittlung des Wissens war bis in die 60er Jahre nicht dem Wissensstand entsprechend und damit waren auch die Auswirkungen der klinischen Anwendung sehr begrenzt. Erst nach dieser Zeit begann sich die Endokrinologie schwerpunktmäßig im Universitätsbereich zu etablieren. Das endokrinologische Verständnis und die Anwendung des Wissens des praktisch tätigen Mediziners blieben unvollkommen. Vielleicht erklärt dies alles auch die in der Öffentlichkeit permanent existierende Furcht vor Hormonen. Eine ganz andere Entwicklung hat sich in den letzten etwa 10–15 Jahren gezeigt. Durch die Vereinfachung der diagnostischen und therapeutischen Maßnahmen und der schnellen Fortentwicklung der Techniken fanden diese sofort Eingang in die Praxis auf breiter Basis. Dabei ist zu berücksichtigen, daß hier der Bereich der Wissenschaft verlassen wird und es um praktische Anwendung geht, bevor die Wissenschaft – soweit überhaupt möglich – Klarheit geschaffen hat über die Konsequenzen.

Von Hippokrates bis
Samuel von Soemmering

Nahezu alles, was wir über die Hypophyse und ihre Hormone wissen, wurde erst in unserem Jahrhundert entdeckt. Aus der Zeit davor gibt es nur fragmentarische Beobachtungen. Die Hypophyse wurde als rudimentäres Organ eingestuft. Die Namensgebung beruht einmal auf der Vorstellung einer Funktion, zum anderen auf den anatomischen Gegebenheiten. *Hippokrates* (̓460 Insel Kos – † 377 v. Chr. in Larissa) war der Meinung, daß die Funktion der Hypophyse darin besteht, Schleim, lateinisch pituita, aus dem Gehirn zu sammeln und durch die Nase auszuscheiden. Nach *Ursula Weiser* sind die Vorstellungen der Hippokratiker über physiologische Prozesse stark spekulativ (in *Engelhardt* u. *Hartmann* 1991). Grundlage ihrer Erklärungen war die Humorallehre. Die Körpersäfte sind die Grundelemente des Menschen. Jedem Saft werden zwei der vier Primärqualitäten zugesprochen.

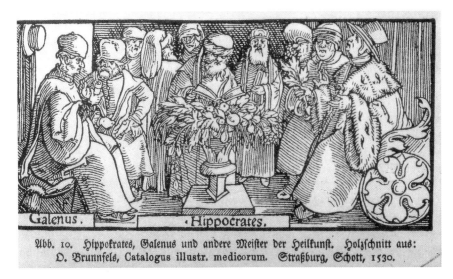

Abb. 10. Hippokrates, Galenus und andere Meister der Heilkunst. Holzschnitt aus: O. Brunnfels, Catalogus illustr. medicorum. Straßburg, Schott, 1530.

Hippokrates, Galen.

Schleim ist kalt-feucht, Blut warm-feucht, gelbe Galle warm-trocken, schwarze Galle kalt-trocken.

Galen (˙129 in Pergamon † 200 in Rom) betrachtete das Interesse an der Anatomie als unentbehrliche Grundlage jeglicher klinischen Tätigkeit. Da die Sektion menschlicher Leichen verpönt war, verwendete er Säugetiere, vor allem Affen und Schweine, von denen er annahm, daß diese dem Menschen am meisten ähneln. Er betrieb die Anatomie vorwiegend unter funktionellen Aspekten und in Verbindung mit physiologischen Fragestellungen. Sein System basierte auf der hippokratischen Tradition. So übernahm *Galen* auch dessen Auffassung über die Hypophyse. Den Hinweis darauf verdanken wir *G. Harris* in seiner Dale Lecture (1971) ‚Humours and Hormones' bei der Besprechung der frühen Beobachtungen zur Hypophysenfunktion. „*Galen* put forward the view that blood ebbed to and for in the carrying ‚vital spirit' to the various organs of the body. ‚Animal spirit' was to be formed from ‚vital spirit' in the brain, with the waste products of this chemical reaction flowing to the base of the brain, down the pituitary stalk and so to the pituitary gland. From this ‚phlegmatic glandule' the waste products were supposed to be passed by ducts through the sphenoid and ethmoid bones to the nasopharynx, where they emerged as ‚pituita or nasal mucus'" (nach *Medvei* 1982). Zur Einordnung dieser Beschreibung sei *Charles Lichtenthaeler* zitiert: „Die galenische Anatomie ist fast nur Tieranatomie. *Galen* beneidet die Frühalexandriner um ihre Sektionen menschlicher Leichen und übernimmt ihr Entdeckungen, sofern er sie für richtig hält. In der vergleichenden Anatomie ist *Galen* Aristoteliker, und er ist es ebenfalls in dem Bestreben, anatomische Forschung mit physiologischen Fragestellungen zu verbinden. Nach seiner Auffassung hängen die Funktionen der Organe stets von deren äußeren Form und innerer Struktur ab. Und für *Galen* wie für den Platonschüler *Aristoteles* ‚tut die Natur nichts umsonst'. Diese natürliche Zweckmäßigkeit versucht der Anatom und Physiologe konsequent herauszustellen. Daß er dabei oft ganz und gar der Spekulation verfällt, liegt auf der Hand . . " (*Lichtenthaeler* 1987).

Der Flame *Andreas Vesalis* (˙1514 in Brüssel – † 1564 Insel Zantos), der erste maßgebliche Anatom der Neuzeit, Professor der Anatomie in Padua, setzte sich mit den Schriften *Galens* intensiv auseinander. *Vesals* Werk „De humani corporis fabrica libri septem" ist mit mehr als 300 Stahlstichen von *Johann Stephan Kalkar*, einem Schüler *Tizians*, ausgestattet. In diesem Werk berichtigte *Vesal* galenische Irrtümer. Aber an der Hippokrates-Galen'schen These zur Hypophyse hielt auch er fest und nannte die Drüse: *Glandula pituitam cerebri excipiens.*

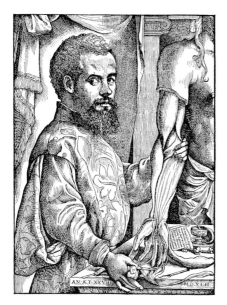

A. *Vesalius* (129 in Pergamon + 200 in Rom).

Conrad Victor Schneider von Wittenberg (1614–1680) widerlegte die Vorstellung, daß es Aufgabe der Hypophyse sei, Schleim oder Phlegma (pituita) des Gehirns durch die Nase auszuscheiden. Er wies nach, daß es keine Verbindung gibt, durch die dies möglich sei. Die bei mazerierten Knochen gefundenen Poren, sind beim Lebenden durch Gefäße verschlossen. Dissertatio de osse cribriformi, et sensu ac organo odoratus (1655) und Liber primus de catarrhis (1660). *Schneider* übte neben seiner Professur in Wittenberg das Amt des Leibarztes des Kurfürsten von Sachsen sowie des Herzogs von Anhalt aus.

Richard Lower (1631–1691) in Oxford vertrat die Meinung, daß Stoffe aus dem Gehirn durch das Infundibulum und den Hypophysenstiel in die Hypophyse gelangen, von wo sie in das Blut abgegeben werden. *Simmer* (1974) hat nachgewiesen, daß es aufgrund eines Übersetzungsfehlers falsch ist, hieraus auf die Annahme einer Hormonbildung zu schließen.

Der Anatom *Samuel Thomas von Soemmering* (1755–1830) prägte den Begriff hypophysis cerebri (1778): Dissertatio de basi encephali et originibus nervorum cranio egredientum libri quinque. Die Dissertation in Göttingen über vergleichende Anatomie des Gehirns, die er seinem Vater widmete, begründete seinen Ruhm als Anatom und Physiologe.

In der deutschsprachigen Literatur hat sich die anatomische Nomenklatur ‚Hypophyse' bis heute durchgesetzt. In englischen Publikationen war

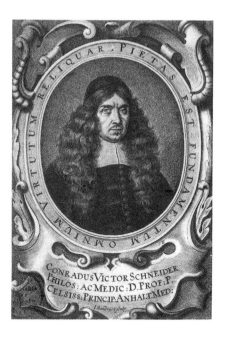

Conrad Victor Schneider (1614–1680):
Professor der Medizin in Wittenberg, Leib-
arzt des Kurfürsten von Sachsen. De catarrhis
1660.

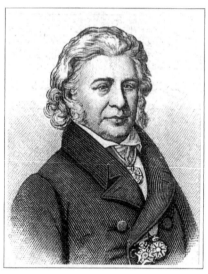

Samuel Thomas von Soemmering (1755–
1830): Anatom und Physiologe in Frankfurt,
1778 Über die Gehirnbasis und die Ursprün-
ge der Gehirnnerven, Lehrbuch vom Bau des
menschlichen Körpers.

dies Anfang des Jahrhunderts auch der Fall. Seit den 30er Jahren wird in diesen jedoch vorwiegend die „Schleim"version benutzt: ‚Pituitary'. Als die vielfältigen Funktionen der Hypophyse immer mehr aufgeklärt wurden, bekamen sie den Namen ‚Meisterdrüse' oder ‚Master Gland'. In der Botanik ist die Hypophyse ein Zellkomplex, der bei der Embryonalentwicklung mancher Pflanzen den Embryo mit dem Embryoträger oder Suspensor verbindet.

Der Name „Gonadotropine" wurde 1930 durch *Wiesner* und *Crew* geprägt. 1938 wurde der Terminus Gonadotropine im Rahmen der 3. Internationalen Konferenz für Standardisierung von Hormonen in Genf als allgemein verbindlich erklärt. *Choh Hao Li* am Hormone Research Laboratory in Berkeley, der den größten Anteil an der chemischen Aufklärung der Hypophysenvorderlappenhormone hat, diskutierte 1962 den Gebrauch des Suffix-tropin oder -trophin. „On the use of -tropin or - trophin in connection with anterior pituitary hormones." „In arriving at final acceptance of terminology for any set of objects or materials or substances coming newly into use after their discovery, a veering course is always steered between the Scylla of logical etymology and the Charybdis of common usage … A good example is furnished by the anterior pituitary hormones, which generically have been called either tropic or trophic hormones, and individually have been designated either -tropins or -trophins, according to geographic location and personal preference. This has been going on now for well over a decade, and practice is still equally divided, with, on the whole, endocrinologists and biochemists, on the other side of the Atlantic preferring the suffix -trophin and those on this continent adhering to tropin; … It is certainly true that usage is a prime determinant of language, but it is our opinion in this laboratory that language must also be used with an awareness of its precise connotations and associations, when these are present; otherwise we are throwing away the real value of meening. For this reason, we have preferred through the years the term tropic to trophic, and the suffix -tropin to -trophin, for these adenohypophyseal hormones, not just on puristic grounds of ‚legitimacy' but on the basis of signification. We feel that the use of one or other of these suffixes is not just an idiosyncratic matter but, rather, that the terminology is intimately connected in this instance with the concept of action of these hormones.

If we review for a moment the derivation of these suffixes, we recall that -tropin comes from the greek tropos, used to denote turning, changing, or tending to turn or change, especially in a specified manner or in response to a specified stimulus, as in heliotropic, isotropic, phototropic. Thus, termino-

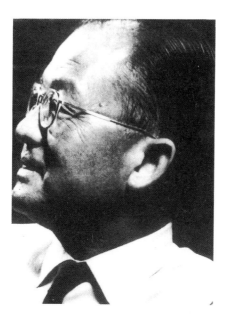

Li, Ch. H. (1913–1987): Seit 1933 in Berkeley. Reinigung, Charakterisierung und Aufklärung der Chemie der Hypophysenvorderlappenhormone und deren Synthese.

logy with this suffix implies the stimulating effect of the hormone on its target organ which is characteristic of all these adenohypophyseal hormones (with, perhaps, the exception of growth hormone, which has not one target organ, although here the soma, the whole body, can be viewed as the ‚target‘ for the hormonal action). The suffix -trophin, on the other hand, derives from the Greek trophé (from trephein, to nourish) and in its combining for denotes nutrition, nourishment, nurture – a meaning which is misleading in the light of our present knowledge of these pituitary hormones.“ (*Stewart* und *Li* 1962).

Anatomie

1838 erschien von *Martin Heinrich Rathke* (1793–1860) in Königsberg „Über die Entstehung der glandula pituitaria". Er nahm an, daß sich die Drüse aus dem Entoderm entwickelt. Man muß sich vergegenwärtigen, daß Dank der Serienfabrikation zuverlässiger Mikroskope etwa um 1830, erst vergleichbare histologische Beurteilungen möglich wurden.

    M. Balfour (1851–1882) wies 1874 und *G. V. Mihalkovics* (1844–1899) 1875 den ektodermalen Ursprung nach. Spätere Untersucher bezweifelten diese Befunde und vermuteten eine Entwicklung sowohl aus dem Ektoderm als auch Entoderm. Die pars anterior wurde 1724 von *Giovanni Domenico Santorini* (1681–1737) beschrieben. Er nannte das milchige Sekret, das er aus dem Gewebe pressen konnte, „glandula pituitaria potior". *T. Lups* publizierte Befunde über die ektodermale Herkunft des Hypophysenvorderlappen und stellte fest, daß eine Zuordnung des Hinterlappen nicht möglich sei (1929). Der Begriff „gonadotrope Hormone" wurde erst 1930 von *Wiesner* und *Crew* geprägt. Der Hinterlappen wurde Neurohypophyse genannt (*H. W. Howell*, 1898). Die spezielle Cytologie der Adenohypophyse geht zurück auf *A. Schönemann* (1892). Er unterschied zwei chromophile Zellklassen: Eosinophile und Cyanophile, später acidophil und basophil genannt (*Mallory*, 1900). *Cushing* (1912) beobachtete eine Differenzierung in chromophobe und chromophile Zellen aufgrund unterschiedlicher Affinität zu Hämatoxylin und Eosin. Die Anfänge der Aufklärung der Beziehung zwischen Struktur und Funktion der Hypophyse werden ausführlich von *R. B. Page* (1988) beschrieben. Durch die Verwendung unterschiedlicher Färbe- und immunhistologischer Methoden erfolgten weitere Differenzierungen (*Romeis*, 1940, *Purves*, 1966, *Page*, 1988). So wurde die Zuordnung der verschiedenen Zelltypen zur spezifischen Hormonbildung möglich. (*Pearse*, 1952, *Pearse* u. *van Noorden*, 1963, *Kracht* und *Hachmeister*, 1969).

Pathologie

Pathologisch-anatomische Veränderungen der Hypophyse wurden zahlreich beschrieben. *Johann Jacob Wepfer* (1620–1695) aus Schaffhausen veröffentlichte 1681 Autopsiebefunde mit einer aufs doppelte vergrößerten Hypophyse. Ähnliche Beobachtungen machten *Théophile Bonet* (1620–1689) und *Raymond Vieussens* (1641–1715). Der Italiener *Andrea Verga* beschrieb 1864 einen Hypophysentumor und 1877 *Vincenzo Brigidi*. *Carl Benda* (1857–1933) konnte zeigen, daß es sich bei einer Akromegalie um einen Eosinophilen-Zell Tumor handelte (1900). Der Pathologe und *Virchow*-Schüler *T. A. E. Klebs* (1834–1913) publizierte zusammen mit *C. F. Fritzsche* 1884 „Zur Pathologie des Riesenwuchses". Der Neurologe an der Salpétrière und *Charcot* Schüler *Pierre Marie* (1983–1940) veröffentlichte 1882 die Befunde von zwei Akromegalie Fällen. Die pathogenetischen Zusammenhänge wurden erst später erkannt. *Wilhelm Rath* publizierte 1888 in seiner Dissertation in Göttingen eine Tabelle von Hypophysentumoren (*Rath* 1888). Funktionelle Veränderungen werden nicht aufgeführt. Auch *Hermann Oppenheim,* der zahlreiche Tumore der Hypophyse beschrieb, schreibt der Hypophyse keine Funktion zu (*Oppenheim* 1898).

In der gleichen Zeit findet man jedoch Einzelbeobachtungen, bei denen ein Zusammenhang zwischen Erkrankungen der Hypophyse und Veränderungen der Gonadenfunktion Erwähnung finden, (siehe bei *Pappenberger,* 1985). Die Kenntnisse über die Funktion der Hypophyse im 19. Jahrhundert beschreibt *Rollestone* in „The endocrine organs in health and disease with an historical review" wie folgt: „The advance of knowledge and the recent elaboration of detail in connexion with endocrine function and disease are best illustrated by the history of the pituitary. Until nearly the beginning of this century it was regarded as little more than a vestigial relic; now it has become the head stone of the corner. In a review of nerve physiology in 1889, it was stated that the pituitary has ‚little, or perhaps no, use in the organism of the higher vertebrates' (TW Shore), and in the same year it was

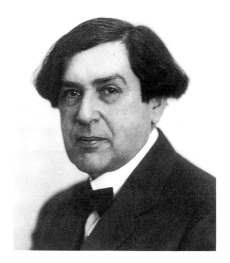

A. Fröhlich (1871–1953): Professor am pharmakologischen Institut in Wien; 1939 Emigration nach Cincinatti. 1901 „Ein Fall von tumor cerebri der Hypophysis ohne Akromegalie", Dystrophia adiposogenitalis. Transnasale Hypophysektomie durch von Eiselsberg.

described as ‚probably the rudiments of an archaic sense organ' (*MacAlister*)" (*Rollestone*, 1936).

Joseph Francois Felix Babinski (1857–1932) ein Schüler von *Charcot*, berichtete im Juni 1900 in der Société de Neurologie in Paris über ein 17jähriges Mädchen mit einem Hypophysentumor (épithélioma) ohne Akromegalie, aber unterentwickelten Genitalorganen.

Alfred Fröhlich (˙1871 Wien – † 1953 Cincinatti/Ohio) hielt 1901 vor der Wanderversammlung des Vereins für Psychiatrie und Neurologie in Wien einen Vortrag mit dem Titel: „Ein Fall von Tumor cerebri der Hypophysis ohne Akromegalie" (1901). Anhand eines von ihm beobachteten Falles und der Literatur beschreibt er die Symptomatik der nach ihm benannten Dystrophia adiposogenitalis. Er verneinte jedoch die bereits von anderen geäußerte Vermutung einer Beziehung zwischen Hypophyse und Gonaden. Bei einem von *Fröhlichs* Patienten, einem 14jährigen Jungen wurde durch *Anton Freiherr von Eiselsberg* (1860–1939), ein Hypophysentumor transnasal entfernt. Sehstörungen und Kopfschmerzen verschwanden und der Patient wurde 56 Jahre alt.

Fröhlich teilte den erfolgreichen Eingriff *Harvey W. Cushing* mit. Beide waren 1901 bei dem Physiologen *Sir Charles Sherrington* (1857–1925) in Liverpool. *Fröhlich* arbeitete bis 1939 in der Pharmakologie in Wien, mußte dann nach dem Einmarsch der Nazis auswandern und ging ans May Institute of Medical Research des Jewish Hospital in Cincinatti.

Bald nach der Entdeckung der Röntgenstrahlen (1895) diagnostizierte *Hermann Oppenheim* bereits 1901 in Berlin eine Vergrößerung der Sella turcica bei einem Patienten mit einem Hypophysentumor. *Arthur Schüller* veröffentlichte 1912 ein Buch über die Röntgendiagnostik mit Beschreibung der Veränderungen der Sella bei Tumoren und des Skeletts bei Akromegalen.

Hypophysen-Chirurgie

Der Londoner Allgemeinchirurg *Sir Victor Horsley* gilt als Pionier der intra-kranialen Operation. 1886 hatte er bei zwei Hunden die Hypophyse ent-fernt. Es werden keine besonderen Symptome beschrieben, nur „that the motor cortex was found to be exceptionally excitable in both animals". 1889 führte er die erste intrakraniale Operation aus. Er publizierte 1906 die Ergebnisse von 10 Craniotomien bei Tumoren der Hypophyse. Durch die Operation, erst auf frontalem, später auf dem temporalen Weg, sollte die durch den Tumor hervorgerufene mechanische Irritation beseitigt und eine Erblindung verhütet werden. Bereits 1893 wurde von *Richard Caton* (1842–1926) und *Frank Paul* (1851–1941) in Liverpool über eine chirur-gische Intervention bei einer Akromegalie berichtet. Die Schmerzen ließen nach, aber der Patient erblindete und verstarb nach 3 Monaten. *Herman Schloffer* (1868–1937) in Innsbruck publizierte 1906 eine Übersicht der verschiedenen Operationsverfahren und führte die erste extrakraniale Opera-

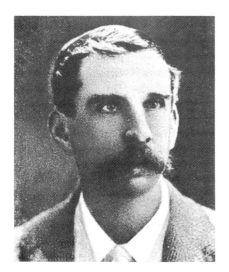

Sir Victor Horsley (1857–1916): Pionier der Neurochirurgie.

tion durch. Als Geburtsstunde der modernen Hirnchirurgie nannte *Harvey Cushing* den 9. Februar 1886, der Tag an dem *Victor Horsley* zum Chirurgen am National Hospital for the Paralysed and Epileptic in London ernannt wurde. *H. Schipperges* bezeichnet *Cushing* als den Schöpfer der modernen Neurochirurgie (*Schipperges* 1995).

Paulesco, Cushing, Aschner

Der Bukarester Physiologe *Nicolas C. Paulesco* (1896–1931) entfernte zusammen mit dem Chirurgen *Balacesco* bei Hunden die Hypophyse auf dem subtemporalen intrakranialen Weg. Die Tiere starben 3 Tage nach der Operation. Hieraus wurde der Schluß gezogen, daß die Hypophyse lebensnotwendig sei (1908). Bei 24 von 52 Hunden und Katzen konnte die vollständige Entfernung mikroskopisch nachgewiesen werden. Die durchschnittliche Überlebenszeit war 24 Stunden. Die Entfernung alleine des Vorderlappens führte zu gleichen Ergebnissen, dagegen die des Hinterlappens zu keinen faßbaren Störungen.

Der Chirurg *Harvey W. Cushing* (˙ 1869 Cleveland/Ohio – † 1939 Boston), in den Hunterian Laboratory of Experimental Medicine der John Hopkins Universität, bestätigte *Paulescos* Befunde (*Crowe, Cushing, Homans*, 1910). Bei über 100 operierten Hunden war die Überlebensrate vor allem

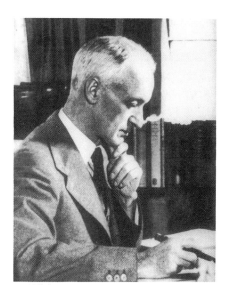

H. Cushing (1869–1939): Schüler des Chirurgen Hallstead am Johns Hopkins Hospital, 1909 „The Hypophysis Cerebri" (hypo-, hyperpituitarism); 1912 Monographie „The pituitary and its disorders". 1932 Cushing Syndrom.

bei jungen Tieren höher. Aber auch *Cushings* Tiere wurden lustlos, zeigten keinen Appetit und verloren an Gewicht bevor sie starben. Wenn nur der Hinterlappen entfernt wurde und die Adenohypophyse intakt blieb, traten die Symptome nicht auf. Dagegen bewirkte die Durchtrennung des Hypophysenstiels die gleichen Symptome wie nach einer Hypophysektomie. In der Publikation „Experimental Hypophysectomy" von 1910 geben *Crowe*, *Cushing* und *Homans* bereits eine historische Übersicht über die bisherigen Hypophysektomie-Versuche. 19 Autoren beginnend 1881 werden aufgelistet, die Methode und die Ergebnisse beschrieben. Die Experimente der Wiener werden in diesem Artikel nicht erwähnt. Im Vordergrund steht die Frage, ob die Hypophyse lebensnotwendig ist oder nicht. Die kritische Analyse zeigt, daß die postoperativen Komplikationen eine erhebliche Rolle spielen. Eine Kontrolle auf die Vollständigkeit der Hypophysektomie erfolgte in nur drei Studien. Vor allem werden die Befunde von *Paulesco* in dieser Arbeit hervorgehoben. „We find, in agreement with *Paulesco,* that a state of apituitarism due to the total removal of the hypophysis leads inevitably to the death of the animal, with a peculiar and characteristic train of symptoms (cachexia hypophyseopriva). ... However, even in the case of adult animals death need not occur after a total removal as promptly as *Paulesco* claimed; whereas puppies may remain in an apparently normal condition for at least 3 weeks before the terminal phenomena appear. ... Definite constitutional disturbances which we may regard as manifestations of hypopituitarism have been observed after partial (anterior lobe) removal in a number of animals kept under observation for long periods of time. The most striking feature is a state of adiposity accompanied by (or resultant to?) a secondary hypoplasia of the organs of generation in adults or a persistence of sexual infantilism in case the primary hypophyseal deficiency antedates adolescence .. ". Durch Transplantationen oder durch Injektion von Extrakten konnte eine Verlängerung der Überlebenszeit erzielt werden. In seinem Vortrag vor der Section or Surgery der American Medical Association in Atlantic City im Juni 1909 „The Hypophysis cerebri Clinical effects of Hyperpituitarism and of Hypopituitarism" verglich *Cushing* die bei den Hunden erhobenen Befunde mit den klinischen Symptomen beim Menschen.

Er differenzierte zwischen Überfunktion, wie bei der Akromegalie und einer Unterfunktion, wie bei Zwergen. Er prägte die Begriffe „hyper- und hypopituitarism", die Kombination beider Zustände nannte er „dyspituitarism" und den völligen Ausfall der Funktion „apituitarism". In einer Anmerkung erläuterte er die Wortschöpfung: „From an etymological point of view the terms *hyper-, hypo-, dys-,* and *a-pituitarism* are doubtless of badly mixed parentage, but there are certain obvious objections to such a combination as *hyperhypophysism*, and I have therefore concluded to retain the Latin word with its Greek prefix. *Hyperpituitism, etc.* might possibly be less unwieldy." Der Vortrag gibt das Wissen um die Hypophyse zu diesem Zeitpunkt eindrucksvoll wieder. „Few chaptesr in the history of medicine tell a more ereditable story than that which relates our progress toward a better understanding of the thyroid and parathyroid glands. …No less satisfactory a tale is in the making as regards a hitherto even more obscure member of the family of ductless glands – the pituitary body – and it is my purpose on this occasion to recount briefly some of the steps already taken toward a better knowledge of the normal function and the part played in certain diseases by this peculiar and inaccessible structure – called ‚l'organe enigmatique' by Van Gehuchten… Regarded by the ancients as an organ which discharged *pituita* or mucus into the nose, and by most scientist of the past century as a mere vestigial relic of prehistoric usefulness, our first insight into a possible functional activity of this gland came from the laboratories of the modern comparative anatomists and embryologists, with many of whom it has been a favorite object of research. …Anatomical studies show us that the pituitary body, present in all vertebrates, is a composite gland with a double source of origin. It is made up (1) of a smaller posterior lobe with a nucleus of neural origin (pars nervosa), which, developing from the infundibular pouch of the thalamencephalon, becomes invested by and intimately fused with a portion of the epithelial sac (pars intermedia) that has arisen from a diverticulum of the buccal epithelium; and (2) of a larger, purely epithelial lobe (pars anterior) arising from the same source as the pars intermedia, from which it remains, however, more or less separated by a cleft – a vestige of the cavity of the original epithelial invagination from the primitive mouth. …The glandular function: There are a number of ways in which we may approach matters relating to the function of a gland: by laboratory methods of comparative physiology, by the experimental production of pathologic conditions, and by observing the symptomatology of clinical cases and correlating them either with postmortem findings or with the conditions disclosed or brought about by surgical procedures…." Nach dem Hinweis auf Paulesco's Untersuchungen fährt Cushing fort, „We have had a number of similar experiences; and indeed believe that we have succeeded in purposefully producing this condition which regard as charactestic of lessened secretion. The adiposity has been associated in some cases with polyuria and transient glycosuria, with shedding of hair, occassionally with unmistakable lessening of sexual activities and even with atrophy of testes and ovaries. …In all these observations,

BULLETIN

OF

THE JOHNS HOPKINS HOSPITAL

Entered as Second-Class Matter at the Baltimore, Maryland, Postoffice.

[Vol. XXI.—No. 230.]   BALTIMORE, MAY, 1910.   Price, 25 Cents

CONTENTS.

EXPERIMENTAL HYPOPHYSECTOMY.[1]

By S. J. CROWE, M. D., HARVEY CUSHING, M. D., and JOHN HOMANS, M. D.

(*From the Hunterian Laboratory of Experimental Medicine, The Johns Hopkins University.*)

I. INTRODUCTION.

The function of one of the so-called ductless glands may be investigated by two principal methods. These may be designated as the positive and the negative methods of studying glandular physiology. The first embraces such procedures as the introduction of the gland or its extracts into the body by feeding or injection in order to produce reactions comparable to those which would be brought about by an exaggeration of the normal glandular activity. By the negative method observations are made upon the effects of lost or diminished function of the gland brought about by its complete or partial experimental removal—conditions therefore simulating grades of hypoactivity.

In the course of our work on the function of the hypophysis many experiments have been made by both of these methods, but the particular object of this paper is to record the results obtained by the indirect or negative method, which should enable us to determine:

(1) Whether the hypophysis, in whole or in part, is necessary for the maintenance of life.

(2) If essential, what symptoms occur antecedent to death.

(3) If not essential to life what effects, if any, are produced by its removal.

(4) Whether after partial removal of the gland definite symptoms supervene in consequence of diminished secretion, and whether a compensatory hypertrophy may occur.

(5) Finally, which of the anatomical subdivisions of the gland is chiefly responsible for the symptoms, if any, which follow the loss or mutilation of the structure as a whole.

In order to secure uncomplicated and trustworthy results by this indirect method of investigating glandular function it is

[1] Certain aspects of our investigations dealing with specific questions have already been published (Effects of Hypophyseal Transplantation Following Total Hypophysectomy in the Canine. *Quart. J. Exper. Physiol.*, 1909, II, No. 4, 389; The Experimental Production of Adipositas Universalis with General Atrophy (Hypopituitarism) to appear in Ziegler's Beiträge) and one of us (Cushing) has advanced some general views on the subject in an attempt to correlate the experimental findings with the clinical phenomena associated with various hypophyseal lesions (The Hypophysis Cerebri: Clinical Aspects of Hyperpituitarism and of Hypopituitarism. *J. Am. M. Ass.*, 1909, LIII, 249. Partial Hypophysectomy for Acromegaly, with Remarks on the Function of the Hypophysis. *Ann. of Surg.*, 1909, L, 1003. The Function of the Pituitary Body. *Am. J. M. Sc.*, 1910, CXXXIX, 473). It is anticipated that further papers dealing with the circulation of the hypophysis, the histologic appearance of the gland associated with varying grades of activity, the alterations of other ductless glands secondary to hypophysectomy; the effects of injection of extract in states of hypopituitarism, and a special discussion of the symptoms of polyuria, glycosuria, etc., will subsequently appear.

popituitarism, possibly the most important thing which we have stumbled upon during our studies of these animals is the occurrence of a thermic response to injections of boiled aqueous emulsion of the pars anterior in cases of anterior lobe deficiency (cf. protocols of *Observations 33 (Table VI)*, *34 (Table VII)*, *54, 55* and *98 (Table VIII)*. This has been repeated without failure in practically all of the later anterior lobe "partials" of our own as well as in those of Dr. Goetsch's series; and judging from a few cases of suspected hypopituitarism in man, it appears to hold true for the human as well— a matter which may prove to be of value for the diagnosis of clinical cases. Needless to say, the reactions were controlled, with negative results, by posterior lobe injections in the partially hypophysectomized animals, as well as by injections of the emulsion of one or the other lobe in normal individuals.

The results given in this paper represent merely a stage in our investigations, and necessarily many suggestive topics have been merely touched upon. Further data in regard to the injection experiments as well as to those with glandular feeding, and a more detailed discussion not only of the histologic appearances of activation in the cells constituting the retained fragments, but also of the post operative alterations in the other ductless glands, must be left for the confirmation and additions of the 1909-1910 experiences.

VI. Summary.

Past investigations have led to no unanimity of opinion in regard to the physiological essentiality of the hypophysis cerebri. Thus, of the two most important studies those of Paulesco favor, while those of Gemelli oppose, the view that loss of the gland is necessarily fatal.

Accurate and uncomplicated removal of the gland from the dog—the animal most suited to these investigations—was impossible before the introduction of Paulesco's subtemporal procedure with its principle of cerebral dislocation, and many of the symptoms described by authors before him must in large part have been due to operative trauma, or, in the absence of symptoms, to incompleteness of removal.

We find, in agreement with Paulesco, that a state of apituitarism due to the total removal of the hypophysis leads inevitably to the death of the animal, with a peculiar and characteristic train of symptoms (cachexia hypophyseopriva). That these symptoms are not due to surgical trauma or post-operative complications is evidenced by the facts (1) that the same operative manipulations leaving the hypophysis in place and omitting the single step of removal leads to no symptoms whatsoever, and (2) that incomplete removals produce no immediate disturbances.

However, even in the case of adult animals death need not occur after a total removal as promptly as Paulesco claimed; whereas puppies may remain in an apparently normal condition for at least 3 weeks before the terminal phenomena appear.

These same symptoms, after the same intervals of time, follow the removal of the entire pars anterior alone, even though the posterior lobe remains in place. On the other hand, removal of the posterior lobe (necessarily leaving a small amount of pars intermedia) not only leads to none of the manifestations of cachexia hypophyseopriva, but does not appear to affect the physiological balance of the animal in any symptomatic way, unless the convulsions and excessive sexual activity which have been seen in a few cases can possibly be ascribed to its absence.

Separation of the hypophyseal stalk, owing to circulatory disturbances is comparable either to a partial hypophysectomy or to a total removal with immediate reimplantation of the excised tissue elsewhere in the body. The gland becomes reattached and the pathways for posterior lobe secretion (supposed to traverse the pars nervosa on its way to the infundibular cavity) may become obstructed by the scar, leading to an accumulation of "hyaline" within the channels of the pars nervosa.

Definite constitutional disturbances which we may regard as manifestations of hypopituitarism have been observed after partial (anterior lobe) removals in a number of animals kept under observation for long periods of time. The most striking feature is a state of adiposity accompanied by (or resultant to?) a secondary hypoplasia of the organs of generation in adults or by a persistence of sexual infantilism in case the primary hypophyseal deficiency antedates adolescence. Polyuria, glycosuria, alterations in the skin and its appendages, (such as œdemas and hypotrichosis) the tendency to a subnormal body temperature, and psychic disturbances are more or less frequent accompaniments—all of them symptoms which occasionally occur with states of adiposity and of sexual infantilism in man, in company with certain pituitary body tumors—states, therefore, which presumably are due to hypophyseal (anterior lobe) deficiency.

Animals, in states of hypopituitarism, appear to have a lowered resistance to infection, exposure or disease, conditions which are apt to precipitate the onset of cachexia hypophyseopriva.

It has been possible, by glandular transplantations or by injections of anterior lobe emulsion, definitely to prolong the life of animals after total hypophysectomy, and likewise to tide over periods of threatened cachexia hypophyseopriva in animals retaining anterior lobe fragments which temporarily may be physiologically insufficient.

Boiled anterior lobe emulsions appear to elicit a characteristic (anaphylactic?) febrile response when injected subcutaneously in states of experimental hypopituitarism.

Crowe, S. J., H. Cushing, J. Homans: Experimental Hypophysectomy. Bull. The John Hopkins Hospital XXI (1910) 127–169.

The Journal of the
American Medical Association

Published under the Auspices of the Board of Trustees

VOLUME LIII	CHICAGO, ILLINOIS, JULY 24, 1909	NUMBER 4

Address

THE HYPOPHYSIS CEREBRI

CLINICAL ASPECTS OF HYPERPITUITARISM AND OF HYPO-
PITUITARISM*

HARVEY CUSHING, M.D.

BALTIMORE

Few chapters in the history of medicine tell a more creditable story than that which relates our progress toward a better understanding of the thyroid and para-thyroid glands. A combination of clinical, experimental and surgical experiences during the past twenty years has served to unveil many of the mysteries which formerly surrounded the function of these structures, whose normal activities prove to be so essential to the maintenance of physiologic equilibrium. Myxedema, cretinism, exophthalmic goiter, surgical myxedema (cachexia strumipriva) and tetany have come to be understandable maladies, definitely amenable to rational methods of treatment—and organotherapy, when glandular activity is subnormal, or partial surgical removal to correct functional over-activity, is a triumph of the experimental method in medicine, at the hands of Horsley, Kocher, Halsted, Gley, Vassale and Generale, Mac-Callum and a host of others.

Not the least memorable incident of the entire story was the recognition, first by the Italian investigators, of the important rôle played by the lesser glands—the parathyroid bodies—in occasioning the so-called acute cachexia thyreopriva with tetanoid symptoms; for without this knowledge the condition of myxedema must have remained obscure from inability to produce its experimental counterpart, and actual investigation of the parathyroids might have been long delayed.

No less satisfactory a tale is in the making as regards a hitherto even more obscure member of the family of ductless glands—the pituitary body—and it is my purpose on this occasion to recount briefly some of the steps already taken toward a better knowledge of the normal function and the part played in certain diseases by this peculiar and inaccessible structure—called "l'organe enigmatique" by Van Gehuchten. Our progress, such as it is, would have been much slower without the previous experiences with the cervical glands, for out of the confusion which long reigned in their case from lack of appreciation of the double glandular rôle a les-

* The Oration on Surgery, read in the Section on Surgery of the American Medical Association, at the Sixtieth Annual Session, held at Atlantic City, June, 1909.

* From an etymological point of view the terms *hyper-*, *hypo-*, *dys-*, and *a-pituitarism* are doubtless of badly mixed parentage, but there are certain obvious objections to such a combination as *hypohypophysism*, and I have therefore concluded to retain the Latin word with its Greek prefix. *Hyperpituitism*, etc., might possibly be less unwieldy.

son has been learned and applied to the pituitary body, for it likewise combines glandular structures of widely differing function.

Not only in view of the general awakening of interest in the subject, but owing to the fact that most of the recent work on the hypophysis has appeared in foreign languages, it has seemed to me that a simple review of our knowledge of the anatomy and physiology of the gland and some discussion necessarily of a more speculative character as to the part it plays in certain diseases would make an appropriate topic for this annual oration.

THE GLANDULAR STRUCTURE

Regarded by the ancients as an organ which discharged *pituita* or mucus into the nose, and by most scientists of the past century as a mere vestigial relic of prehistoric usefulness, our first insight into a possible functional activity of this gland came from the laboratories of the modern comparative anatomists and embryologists, with many of whom it has been a favorite object of research. As a knowledge of its structure, development and morphologic significance is essential to the proper understanding of matters relating to its function, it may not be out of place to briefly recall here some few of the more important facts:

Rathke, in 1838, described an invagination of mucous membrane, supposedly arising from the anterior end of the foregut—since known as Rathke's pouch—and correctly attributed to this origin the epithelial portion of the pituitary body, which before this time was thought to be wholly derived from the brain. It remained for Götte and Balfour and Mihalkovics, in 1874 and 1875, to show that the invagination described by Rathke was derived from the embryonic buccal cavity rather than from the primitive gut, and hence was of ectodermic rather than of entodermic origin.

This ectodermic and epithelial pouch of Rathke, therefore, projecting from the buccal cavity and pressing against the floor of the anterior cerebral vesicle, leads to a downward fold in its wall, which becomes the early infundibulum. The stalk of the epithelial pouch becomes cut off, leaving a closed sac—the hypophyseal sac—which embraces the thickening wall or infundibular body at the tip of the vesicular fold, and the combined epithelial and nervous structure represents the anlage of the adult hypophysis. As the primitive gland develops further the epithelium of the anterior or lower part of the closed sac representing the remains of Rathke's pouch becomes thickened, forming the anterior lobe of the pituitary body. A more or less definite cleft separates this portion of the gland from the so-called posterior lobe, composed of the upper portion of the primitive closed epithelial sac together with the infundibular body to which it has become intimately adherent and with which it remains functionally associated. It is the persistence of this cleft in the mammalian hypophysis which usually permits of an easy, gross anatomic or surgical separation of the two lobes.

Thus the neural portion of the gland (the infundibular body) becomes surrounded by an intimate epithelial investment pos-

Cushing, H.: The Hypophysis Cerebri. Clinical aspects of hyperpituitarism and of hypopituitarism. J. Am. med. Ass. LIII (1909) 249–255.

not only on the hypophysis cerebri, but on any other of the ductless glands, there is one vitally important matter that is not to be disregarded – namely, the close physiologic interrelation of all these structures. It is impossible to remove – probably partially to remove – the hypophysis without producing marked alterations in all other glands – thyroid, parathyroid, adrenal, testicle, ovaries, islands of Langerhans, and thymus…" Bei der Besprechung der klinischen Symptomatologie bezieht sich Cushing auf Fröhlich, Marie, von Eiselsberg und eigene Beobachtungen. „Two conditions, one due to a pathological increased activity of the pars anterior of the hypopysis (hyperpituitarism), the other to a diminished activity of the same epithelial structure (hypopituitarism) seem capable of clinical differentation. the former express itself chiefly as a process of overgrowth – gigantism, when originating in youth, acromegaly when originating in adult life. The latter expresses itself chiefly as an excessive, often a rapid, deposition of fat with persistence of infantile sexual characteristics when the process dates from youth, and a tendency toward a loss of the acquired signs of adolescence, when it first appeared in adult life" (Cushing 1909).

1910 wurde Cushing, nach seiner Ausbildung bei William Stewart Halstead am Johns Hopinks Hospital, Surgeon-in-Chief und Professor der Harvard Medical School und 1912 bis 1932 Surgeon-in-Chief am Peter Brent Brigham Hospital. Neben der Monographie „The Pituitary Body and its Disorders" (1912), erschien 1932 „Intracranial Tumours" mit der Beschreibung von 2000 Fällen. „Die Entwicklung der Hirnchirurgie" von Schipperges (1955) und das Kapitel 'Pituitary' in Welbourne, The History of Endocrine Surgery (1990) geben eine detaillierte historische Übersicht.

Bernhard Aschner (*1883 Wien–† 1960 New York), Operationszögling an der Wiener Universitätsklinik für Chirurgie bei A. Freiherr von Eiselsberg, verbesserte die Technik der Hypophysektomie, indem er den transbukkalen Zugang wählte. Er hatte beobachtet, daß die häufigste Todesursache bei dem bis dahin benutzten transzerebralen Zugang, die Verletzung des Circulus arteriosus Willisii war. Es gelang Aschner bei jungen Hunden die Hypophyse total zu entfernen und die Tiere überlebten (1909). Er beobachtete einen Wachstumsstillstand und eine Hypoplasie der Genitalorgane.

Im Archiv für Gynäkologie erschien 1912 die Arbeit: ‚Über die Beziehungen zwischen Hypophyse und Genitale.': „Es wurden von mir im ganzen 88 Tiere operiert, und zwar teils mittels totaler Exstirpation der Hypophyse, teils isolierter Exstirpation des Vorder- oder Hinterlappens oder endlich mittels partieller Exstirpation des Vorderlappens." Er beschreibt erstmals eine ovarielle und uterine Atrophie nach isolierter Schädigung des Zwischenhirns

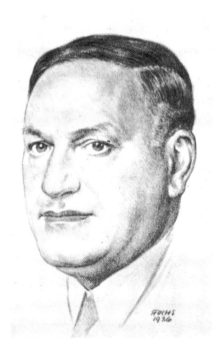

Aschner, B. (1883–1960): Assistent bei dem Chirurgen A. Freiherr von Eiselsberg und bei dem Gynäkologen Friedrich Schauta in Wien. Untersuchungen zur Funktion der Hypophyse durch Hypophysektomie auf bukkalem Weg. 1911 zus. mit Grigoriu Nachweis einer laktogenen Wirkung von Plazentaextrakten; 1912 Entdeckung der Beziehung zwischen Hypothalamus und Gonaden. 1939 Emigration nach New York.

unter Schonung der Hypophyse. In der 127 Seiten umfassenden Publikation berichtet Aschner seine Befunde bei 80 Hunden, von denen 63 komplett hypophysektomiert waren. Die Ausfallserscheinungen waren besonders ausgeprägt bei den jungen Tieren. Eine weitere Arbeit unterteilt in fünf Kapitel erscheint im gleichen Jahr in Pflüger's Archiv für die gesamte Physiologie des Menschen und der Tiere: 'Über die Funktion der Hypophyse'. Im 1. Kapitel gibt Aschner eine kritische Analyse der bisherigen Exstirpationsversuche an der Hypophyse. Ausführlich setzt er sich mit Paulescos Experimenten auseinander. „Paulesco gelangt aufgrund aller seiner Versuche zu folgendem Resumée: 1. Die totale Hypophysenexstirpation hat in kurzer Zeit den Tod des Tieres zur Folge. Die mittlere Lebensdauer ist 24 Stunden. 2. Wenn die Tiere die Operation längere Zeit überleben, so handelt es sich um partielle oder fast totale Hypophysenexstiraption. 3. Der Ausfall der Hypophyse nach der partiellen oder fast totalen Exstiraption hat keine charakteristischen Symptome zur Folge; auch bei längerem Überleben hat Paulesco in seinen Versuchen keine trophische Störungen beobachtet. 4. Die vollständige Abtragung des Vorderlappens kommt der totalen Hypophysenexstirpation gleich. 5. Die Entfernung des Nervenlappens macht keine Störungen. 6. Die Abtrennung

(Aus dem k. k. Institute für allgem. und experim. Pathologie der Universität Wien.)

Über die Funktion der Hypophyse.

Von

Dr. **Bernhard Aschner.**

(Mit 47 Textfiguren und Tafel I.)

Inhaltsübersicht.

Aschner, B.: Über die Funktion der Hypophyse, Pflügers Arch. für Physiologie 146 (1912) 1–146.

der Hypophyse von der Hirnbasis ist tödlich. 7. Daraus wird gefolgert, daß die Hypophyse ein zum Leben unentbehrliches Organ ist, dessen Entfernung rasch zu Tode führt. Von seinen Teilen ist der Drüsenlappen der funktionell wichtige Anteil". Bei Cushing bezieht sich Aschner auf dessen Vortrag 1909 auf dem internationalen Kongreß in Budapest und frühere Arbeiten. Cushing habe eine ähnliche Methode wie Paulesco benutzt. „Daß die Operationsmethode Cushings gewiß keine empfehlenswerte sein kann, geht schon daraus hervor, daß es ihm unter hundert Fällen nur fünfmal gelungen ist, trophische Störungen zu erzeugen". „Cushings beibehaltenes Resumée, daß die Hypophyse ein absolut lebenswichtiges Organ darstelle, erscheint durch die zitierten Arbeiten wohl nicht völlig eindeutig bewiesen". Im 2. Kapitel beschreibt Aschner die eigene Methodik der Versuche und deren Ergebnisse. Die Exstirpation, die minutiös beschrieben wird, erfolgte auf dem bukkalen Zugang, „Die ganze Operation dauert in der Regel eine Stunde". 63 totale und 16 partielle Exstirpationen an Hunden wurden durchgeführt, 50 Hunde dienten als Kontrollen. Die Befunde werden detailliert beschrieben. „All diese trophischen Störungen werden in gleicher Weise durch die Exstirpation der ganzen Hypophyse, ebenso wie durch die Exstirpation des Vorderlappens allein hervorgerufen." In einem Anhang zu diesem Kapitel erwähnt Aschner die Wirkung von Hypophysenfütterung, Extraktinjektionen und Transplantationen. Eigene Fütterungsversuche mit Hypophysentabletten an einem 16 Jahre alten hypoplastischen menschlichen Zwerg ergaben eine Wachstumszunahme von 7 cm in 5 Monaten. Im 3. Kapitel über den Stoffwechsel der hypophysipriven Tiere ist der Abschnitt über die Beziehungen der Hypophyse zu den übrigen Blutdrüsen besonders zu beachten. Aschner bezieht sich auf das von Eppinger, Falta und Rudinger (1908) aufgestellte Schema über die Wechselwirkung zwischen Thyroidea, Pankreas, Chromaffinen System und Epithelkörperchen. Er fügt in dieses Schema die Hypophyse und die Keimdrüsen ein. Im 4. Kapitel geht es um die Funktion des Infundibulum und tuber cinereum und deren Bedeutung für die Physiologie und Pathologie der Hypophyse. Bei Zerrung oder Durchtrennung des Hypophysenstiels, Reizung des Tuber cinereum, kommt es zu Veränderungen von Puls, Blutdruck und Atmung. Damit ist für Aschner auch geklärt, daß die Verletzung des Tuber cinereum die Ursache des Mißlingens in Versuchen früherer Autoren ist. „Damit ist auch die Frage von der absoluten Lebenswichtigkeit der Hypophyse endgültig im negativen Sinne entschieden." Im 5. Kapitel wird die Anwendung auf die menschliche Pathologie besprochen. Nach historischem Überblick werden die Akromegalie, die Dysplasia adiposogenitalis, Zwergwuchs und Infantilismus, der Riesenwuchs, an-

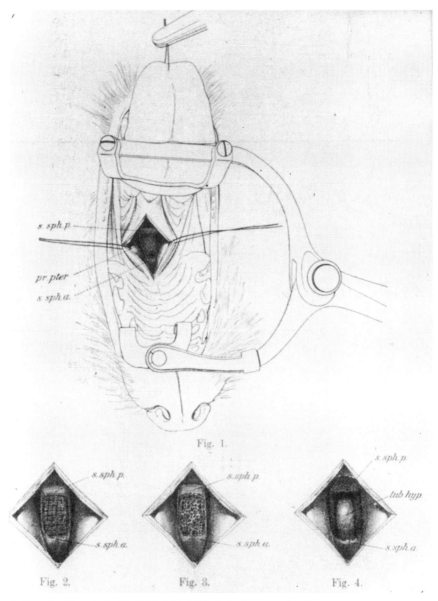

Fig. 1.

Fig. 2.   Fig. 3.   Fig. 4.

Aschner, B.: Pflüger's Archiv 1912 S. 24: 1) Technik der Hypophysektomie.

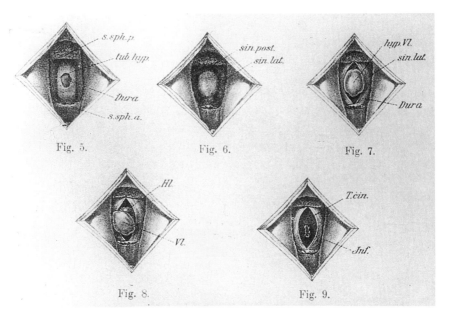

Fig. 5. Fig. 6. Fig. 7.

Fig. 8. Fig. 9.

In der Mitte der lichten Vorwölbung der Lamina externa (Hypophysenwulst) wird mittels der Meiselspitze ein kleines Loch angebracht (Abb. 5), wodurch die weiße Dura mater zum Vorschein kommt. Von diesem Loch aus wird mittels eines sehr feinen scharfen Löffels die papierdünne Lamina interna nach Art einer Eierschale rings herum so weit abgetragen, bis die venösen Sinusse hinten und an beiden Seiten deutlich blosgelegt sind. Am vorderen Ende konfluieren die Sinusse nicht, sondern lassen einen kleinen Zwischenraum frei, vor welchem das Chiasma liegt. Nun wird wieder mit Alkohol ausgetupft und hierauf mit einem sehr spitzen Messer das zwischen den Sinussen gelegene Feld der Dura mater median gespalten, ohne die Sinusse zu verletzen. Es fließt dabei Liquor cerebrospinalis aus, und der gelbrötliche Vorderlappen der Hypophyse tritt aus der Duralöffnung hervor.

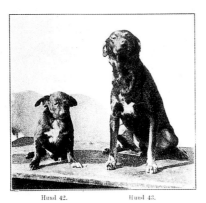

Hund 42. Hund 43.

Fig. 17. Hund 42 und 43 im Alter von 12 Monaten.

S. 39, Abb. 17. Hypophysektomierter Hund und Kontrolltier aus dem gleichen Wurf, demonstriert auf dem Physiologenkongress September 1910 in Wien.

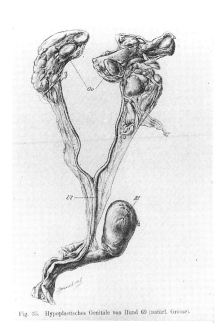
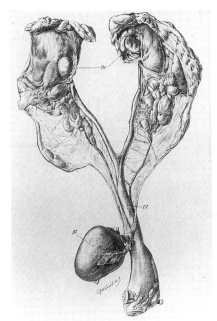

Fig. 35. Hypoplastisches Genitale von Hund 69 (natürl. Grösse).

Fig. 36. Normales weibl. Genitale von Hund 70 (natürl. Grösse).

S. 57, Abb. 35. Hypoplastisches Genitale, Hund 69, im Alter von 3 Monaten Exstirpation der Hypophyse, im Alter von 4 Monaten getötet. Genitale entspricht dem eines ca. 3 Monate alten Hundes.
S. 58 Abb. 36. Normales weibliches Genitale, virginelles, geschlechtsreifes Kontrolltier.

dere Wachstumsstörungen und Blutdrüsenerkrankungen, sowie die Beziehungen zwischen Hypophyse und Genitale abgehandelt. „Das die Hypophyse in vielfacher Wechselbeziehungen zu allen innersekretorischen Drüsen des Körpers steht, geht aus vielen experimentellen und klinischen Tatsachen hervor; besonders innig sind diese Beziehungen zu den Keimdrüsen... Die besprochenen morphologischen Veränderungen der Hypophyse sind der Vergrößerung der Schilddrüse, der Nebenniere, ferner analogen Veränderungen der Leber, des Pankreas, der Epithelkörperchen, der Milz und des Corpus luteum in der Gravidität analog zu setzen." Den Abschluß dieser grundlegenden Publikation bildet ein Literaturverzeichnis von über 500 Zitaten (Aschner, 1912). Im gleichen Jahr erscheint auch die Arbeit „Zur Physiologie des Zwischenhirns", in der Aschner erstmals eine ovarielle und uterine Atrophie nach isolierter Schädigung des Zwischenhirns beschreibt.

Aschner war von 1904 bis 1907 Demonstrator am Anatomischen Institut in Wien, ein Jahr Operationszögling bei Anton Freiherr von Eiselsberg in

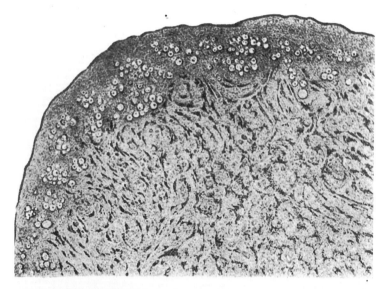

Fig. 37. Schnitt durch das hypoplastische Ovarium von Hund 69.

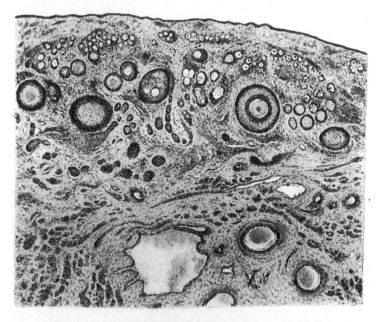

Fig. 38. Schnitt durch das normale Ovarium von Hund 70.

S. 59 Abb. 37 u. 38. Schnitt durch das hypoplastische Ovar von Hund 69 und das normale von Hund 70.

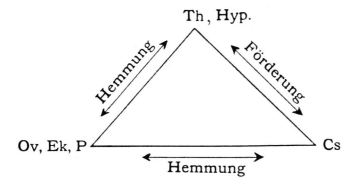

Th , Hyp.

Hemmung

Förderung

Ov, Ek, P

Cs

Hemmung

Aschners Schema zur hemmenden und fördernden Wirkung der innersekretorischen Drüsen.

der Chirurgie und ab 1908 an der Frauenklinik bei Friedrich Schauta. Neben seiner klinischen Ausbildung machte er seine wissenschaftlichen Untersuchungen bei dem Pathologen Richard Paltauf. 1918 erschien 'Die Blutdrüsenerkrankungen des Weibes und ihre Beziehungen zur Gynäkologie'und 1924 Handbuchartikel über Beziehungen der Drüsen mit innerer Sekretion zum weiblichen Genitale. Als Halbjude mußte er 1939 Wien verlassen. Er wurde Chief of the Outpatient Department an der Stuyvesant Clinic in New York. Sein ursprüngliches Arbeitsgebiet setzte er nicht fort. Aschner hat die Werke Paracelsus ins Deutsche übersetzt.

Die Entwicklung der Erkenntnisse über die Hypophysenfunktion in der Zeit von 1908–1912 hat Cushing in seinem schon erwähnten Vortrag „The hypophysis cerebri" zusammengefaßt.

Der Prosektor des Instituts für Pathologische Anatomie des Stadthausspitals in Lainz bei Wien, Jacob Erdheim (*1874 Boryslaw/Galizien–1937 Wien), beobachtete die Veränderungen der Hypophyse in der Schwangerschaft (1909): Vergrößerung des Vorderlappens und die Bildung großer eosinophiler Zellen, den sog. Schwangerschaftszellen. Die Größenzunahme der Hypophyse war erstmals 1898 von L. Comte beschrieben worden (Comte, 1898). Die Größenzunahme nach Kastration bei beiden Geschlechtern wurde von Tandler und Grosz entdeckt (Tandler u. Grosz, 1907, 1908). Von Erdheim stammt auch die Beschreibung der Kraniopharyngiome (Erdheim Tumor, 1904), des hypophysären Zwergwuchs, sowie der nanosomia pituitaria (1916). Den ersten Bericht einer multiplen endokrinen Drüsenerkrankung verdanken wir auch Erdheim. Bei einer Autopsie eines Akromegalen fand er nicht nur eine vergrößerte Hypophyse, sondern gleichzeitig auch eine diffuse Struma, vergrößerte Nebenschilddrüsen und eine Pankreasnekrose.

Hypophysen-Vorderlappeninsuffizienz

Der Pole *L. K. Glinski* publizierte 1913 sowohl in einer polnischen Zeitschrift als auch in der Deutschen Medizinischen Wochenschrift erstmals über 2 Fälle mit einer post partum Nekrose des Hypophysenvorderlappen.

Morris Simmonds (1855–1925), erst praktischer Arzt in Hamburg, dann Prosektor im Krankenhaus St. Georg berichtete am 6. Januar 1914 im Ärztlichen Verein über einen Fall einer Hypophysennekrose, die 11 Jahre nach einer Puerperalsepsis mit nachfolgender Amenorrhö zum Tode führte. Die einzige Angabe bei der Einlieferung in die Pathologie war, „daß sie vor 2 Tagen allmählich besinnungslos geworden sei ... ." *Simmonds* beschreibt das Resultat der Sektion: „So hätte auch die Sektion keine Aufklärung gebracht, wenn ich nicht zum Schluß den Hirnanhang herausgenommen hätte. Sofort fielen die kleinen Dimensionen, die schlaffe Konsistenz, das völlig abnorme Aussehen des nur 0,3 g wiegenden Organs auf. Die mikroskopische Untersuchung war überraschend. Von der Neurohypophyse war überhaupt nichts

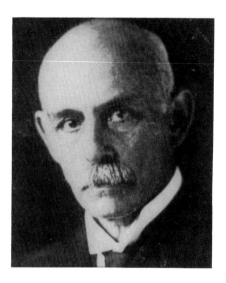

M. Simmonds (1855–1925): (Staatsarchiv Hamburg.) Praktischer Arzt und Prosektor am Allgemeinen Krankenhaus St. Georg in Hamburg. 1914 erste Beschreibung einer postpartalen Hypophysenvorderlappen-insuffizienz.

Aus dem Allgemeinen Krankenhause St. Georg in Hamburg.

Ueber Hypophysisschwund mit tödlichem Ausgang.[1)]

Von Prof. M. Simmonds.

M. H.! Es gibt für den Pathologischen Anatomen nichts Unbehaglicheres, als wenn er am Schlusse einer Sektion eingestehen muß, daß er weder Krankheit noch Todesursache erkannt hat. Er wird jedes Organ noch einmal prüfen, er wird an der Hand der klinischen Daten noch einmal alle Möglichkeiten erwägen, um doch schließlich mit einem „non liquet" sich zu bescheiden. Zum Glück kommen solche Vorkommnisse auch bei einem großen Material nur selten vor.

Vor wenigen Wochen glaubte ich wieder vor einem solchen „non liquet" zu stehen.

Eine 46 jährige Frau war in besinnungslosem Zustande ins Krankenhaus gebracht worden mit der einzigen Angabe, daß sie vor zwei Tagen allmählich besinnungslos geworden sei und sich aus diesem Zustande nicht wieder erholt habe. Auf der Abteilung des Herrn Kollegen Saenger wurde eine äußerst sorgfältige Untersuchung ausgeführt — ohne Erfolg. Urin war zucker- und eiweißfrei, das Lumbalpunktat von normaler

Ist diese sicherlich gut fundierte Voraussetzung aber richtig, so liegen die Verhältnisse klar vor, und der Krankheitsverlauf ist kurz der: Eine bis dahin gesunde Frau erkrankt an schwerer Puerperalsepsis. Sie erleidet eine septische Nekrose des Hirnanhangs. Infolge des Verlustes dieses lebenswichtigen Organs treten schwere Ausfallserscheinungen: Menopause, Muskelschwäche, Schwindel und Bewußtlosigkeitsanfälle, Anämie, rasches Altern, kurzum, ein „Senium praecox" ein. Die restierenden intakten Drüsenfragmente atrophieren allmählich in dem umgebenden Bindegewebe. Das Organ wird absolut insuffizient, die Frau geht im Koma zugrunde. Die Sektion ergibt als einzige Todesursache einen fast totalen Schwund der Hypophysis.

[1)] Vorgetragen im Aerztlichen Verein in Hamburg am 6. Jan. 1914.

Simmonds, M.: Über Hypophysisschwund mit tödlichem Ausgang. DMW 40 (1914) 322–328 (Genehmigung G. Thieme Verlag, Stuttgart).

mit Sicherheit zu erkennen. Von der pars intermedia nur ganz vereinzelte, kleine, koloidhaltige Zysten. Von den drüsigen Vorderlappen waren nur ganz einzelne Zellzüge oder minimale runde Häufchen erhalten geblieben. Nach diesen Befunden war eine hochgradige Atrophiebildung der Hypophyse zu diagnostizieren, und da wir durch die zahllosen publizierten Tierexperimente wissen, daß der Hirnanhang ein absolut lebenswichtiges Organ ist, daß eine Entfernung beim Tier in mehr oder minder langer Zeit unter den Erscheinungen von Asthenie und schließlich von Koma zum Tode führt, war dieser Hypophysenschwund als Todesursache in unserem Fall zu bezeichnen" (*Simmonds*, 1914). Aus der Krankenakte ging hervor, daß die Frau 11 Jahre vorher mit 36 Jahren nach der Geburt des letzten Kindes eine schwere Puerperalsepsis hatte, nie wieder menstruierte, schwach und matt wurde, abmagerte und vorzeitig alterte.

Weitere Beobachtungen einer „hypophysären Kachexie" folgten. *Simmonds* erkannte als Ätiologie der Zerstörung der Hypophyse durch embolische Prozesse mit Nekrosebildung, aber auch andere Veränderungen, wie ein Tumor oder eine Tuberkulose. Trotz der von ihm gewählten Bezeichnung, betonte *Simmonds*, daß die Kachexie nicht obligat sei. *L. Lichtwitz*, Internist am Allgemeinen Krankenhaus Altona, beschrieb 1922 drei weitere Fälle und schlug vor, die Erkrankung als „Simmond'sche Krankheit" zu bezeichnen.

Edgar Reye (1882–1945), Oberarzt der IV. medizinischen Abteilung des Universitäts Krankenhaus Eppendorf, beschrieb 1926 das klassische Bild

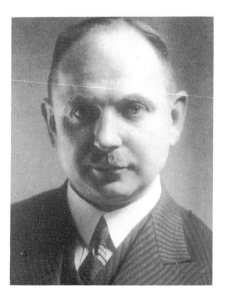

E. Reye (1882–1945): Internist am Universitätskrankenhaus Eppendorf und Allgemeinen Krankenhaus Barmbeck in Hamburg. 1926 Beschreibung einer postpartalen Hypophysenvorderlappeninsuffizienz.

einer Hypophysenvorderlappen-Insuffizienz als Folge einer postpartalen Blutung. *Reye* empfahl, wie vor ihm schon *Lichtwitz,* die Diagnose „Simmond'sche Krankheit" nur dann zu stellen, wenn sich bei einem Ausfall der Hypophysenfunktion eine Kachexie entwickelt. Er widersprach *Simmonds* Auffassung, daß eine Sepsis Vorbedingung für die Zerstörung der Hypophyse sei. Komplizierte Entbindungen oder postpartale Blutungen seien die Ursache. „Noch einmal hebe ich ganz kurz das Wichtigste aus der fast monotonen Anamnese und aus dem mehr oder weniger rasch sich entwickelnden Symptomenbild, wie es sich aus allen meinen Erfahrungen ergibt, hervor: Schwere Entbindung, starker Blutverlust, langes Krankenlager, (keine Sepsis), Ausfallen der Menses, Erlöschen der Libido, Fettansatz, zunehmende körperliche Schwäche, und geistige Schwerfälligkeit, Blaßwerden der Haut, Ausfallen der Haare und der Zähne, Übertemperatur, Frostgefühl, Magendarmstörungen, Eosinophilie, niedriger Blutdruck, Herabsetzung des Grundumsatzes, Kachexie. Selbstverständlich dabei auch Atrophie aller übrigen Blutdrüsen" (*Reye* 1928). Bereits in der ersten Publikation 1926 erwähnt *Reye* die Therapie mit „Vorderlappensubstanz" der Fa. *Passek* und *Wolf,* Hamburg. „Wie ich bei allen meinen drei Fällen erproben konnte, wirkt Praephyson sowohl als Injektion als bei Verfolgung per os." 1928 bestätigte er dies: „Der Erfolg der Therapie ist überraschend schnell und ganz besonders erfreulich. Ein 2 ½ Jahre kranker und kaum brauchbarer Mensch in wenigen Wochen sympto-

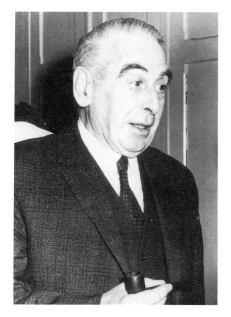

H. L. Sheehan (1900 – 1988): Praktischer Arzt in Carlisle, Lecturer in Pathology, Director of Research in Glasgow, 1946 Professor in Liverpool. 1937 „Post partum necrosis of the anterior pituitary".

616.831.43—002.4 : 618.6

POST-PARTUM NECROSIS OF THE ANTERIOR PITUITARY.

H. L. SHEEHAN.

From the Research Department, Glasgow Royal Maternity Hospital.

(PLATES XXXIII.-XXXVI.)

 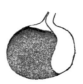

FIG. 1.— Pituitary of case I ; sagittal section. Black = area of necrosis.

FIG. 2. — Pituitary of case II ; sagittal section.

FIG. 3.—Pituitary of case III ; sagittal section. Tiny focus of necrosis only.

Sheehan, H. L.: Post-partum necrosis of the anterior pituitary. J. Pathol. Bacteriol. 45 (1937) 189–214.

matisch völlig geheilt! ... ein so schöner und absolut beweisender Erfolg, daß sogar die Menses wieder auftraten..."

1937 erschien die Publikation von *Harold L. Sheehan* (1900–1988), Pathologe an der Universität Liverpool, „Post partum necrosis of the anterior pituitary". Bei 59 Autopsien von Wöchnerinnen hatte *Sheehan* in sieben Fällen eine komplette Nekrose der Adenohypophyse gefunden und viermal geringere Zerstörungen. „The fully developed lesion is a coagulative necrosis with the typical appearances of an infarct and an ischaemic origin appears to be the most reasonable explantation on general pathological grounds" (*Sheehan,* 1937). *A. Jores* schlug vor die postpartale Hypophyseninsuffizienz „Reye-Sheehan-Syndrom" zu nennen (*Jores,* 1955).

Evans, Smith, Aschheim, Zondek

In den ersten Jahrzehnten unseres Jahrhunderts häuften sich die Befunde, daß die Funktion der Geschlechtsorgane durch einen extragonadalen Faktor gesteuert wird. Bis dahin war die Hypophyse als ein rudimentäres Relikt eingestuft worden. Die tierexperimentellen und klinischen Beobachtungen wurden zur Grundlage der weiteren Entwicklung.

1922 berichteten *Evans* und *Long* in der National Academy of Science, daß sie mit der Verabreichung von Extrakten aus Ochsen-Hypophysen bei Ratten eine Steigerung des Wachstums und eine Luteinisierung erzielten (*Evans* u. *Long,* 1921, 1922). Das Gewebe wurde im Mörser zerkleinert, in Lockes Lösung aufgeschwemmt, dekantiert und injiziert. 1924 faßte *Evans* in seiner Harvey Lecture zusammen: „We may nevertheless be certain: firstly, that the anterior hypophysis is indispensable for growth to adult stature, a lessened amount of its hormone being the direct cause of an important group of endocrine dystrophies, and an increased amount of the hormone being the direct cause of overgrowth. Secondly, the hypophysis stands in ne-

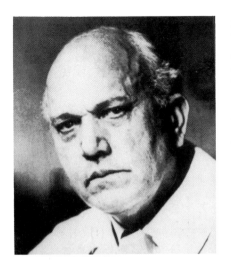

Evans, H. Mc. (1882–1971) (*R. O. Greep*): Entwickelte zusammen mit J. A. Long durch Kreuzung von Wistar Ratten mit wilden grauen Ratten den Long-Evans Stamm, den Farbstoff Evans Blue; beschrieb den Estruszyklus der Ratte; entdeckte Vitamin E und dessen chemische Struktur; 1921 isolierte er das erste aktive Prinzip des Hypophysenvorderlappen, Wachstumshormon. Evans wurde „Master of the Maser Gland" und „Mister Antepituitarism" genannt.

cessary relationship to normal function of the thyroid, sex glands and adrenal cortical tissue" (*Evans,* 1924).

Herbert LcLean Evans (˙ 1882 Modesto/Californien – † 1971 Berkeley/Californien) hatte bei *Paul Ehrlich* in Frankfurt, sowie bei dem Chemiker *Schulemann* und dem Chirurgen *E. E. Goldmann* in Freiburg gearbeitet. 1915 wurde er Chairman in Anatomy der University of California. Er wurde genannt „Master of the Master Gland" oder „Mister Antepituitarism". Zusammen mit *Joseph A. Long* erkannte er die Bedeutung eines standardisierten Tierstammes: Long-Evans Ratten. „*Evans* became world famous for his pioneering work at Berkeley in endocrinology, reproductive physiology, and nutrition. When *Evans* began his work at Berkeley, only two hormones were available to the clinician, thyroid hormone and epinephrine. ... This manyfaced man with his extravagantly diverse interests was truly a giant in endocrinology and a revolutionary in biomedical research who lived life to the hilt, but whose personal qualities stirred people up and made enemies" (*Grumbach,* 1982).

1916 berichtete *Philip E. Smith* über die Entfernung des epithelialen Anteils der Hypophyse bei Kaulquappen, die zur Retardierung der gonadalen Entwicklung führte (*Smith,* 1916). *Benett Allen* im Department of Zoology, University of Kansas machte ähnliche Beobachtungen, die Schilddrüse wurde

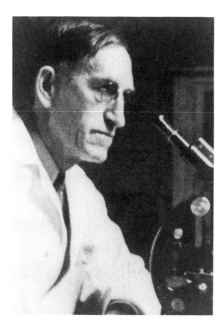

Smith, Philip E. (1884–1970): University of California in Berkeley. Perfektionierte die parapharyngeale Hypophysektomie; 1930: „Hypophysektomie and replacement therapy".

atrophisch und die Metamorphose blieb aus. Die Erscheinungen konnten durch Transplantation von Froschhypophysen behoben werden (*B. Allen,* 1916, 1920). Zusammen mit *Th. Engle* konnte *Smith* mit Hypophysen Homo-Transplantaten bei Ratten und Mäusen eine vorzeitige sexuelle Reifung induzieren (1927). Voraussetzung für diese Versuche war eine komplette Hypophysektomie bei juvenilen Tieren. *Smith* beherrschte die Technik, die Tiere überlebten mehrere Monate. Es kam zum Wachstumsstillstand, zur Atrophie der Gonaden, Schilddrüse, Nebenschilddrüse und Nebennierenrinde. Die Tiere entwickelten ein Syndrom vergleichbar der Simmond'schen Kachexie beim Menschen. „Hypophysectomy in the rat gives an invariable syndrome, the main features of which are: an almost complete inhibition of growth in the young animal, and a progressive loss of weight (cachexia) in the adult; an atrophy of the genital system with loss of libido sexualis, and in the female an immediate cessation of the sex cycles; an atrophy of the thyroids, parathyroids, and suprarenal cortex; and a general physical impairment characterized by a lowered resistance to operative procedures, loss of appetite, weakness and a flabbiness that readily distinguishes the hypophysectomised from the normal animal. It seems unlikely that they can live a normal life span. Attempts carried on for the last 3 years to secure a successful replacement therapy have proved successful as regards all the disabilities arising from the hypophysectomy only when the fresh living hypophyseal tissue was administered" (*Smith,* 1927).

Philip Edward Smith war Anatom in Berkeley, Stanford und an der Columbia University. „*Smith* was a modest, silent, shy but kindly man, who developed an exceptional skill in hypophysectomy in the tadpole and the rat" (*Medvei,* 1982). Zur gleichen Zeit beobachteten *Selmar Aschheim* und *Bernhard Zondek* an der Universitätsfrauenklinik der Charité in Berlin, daß Implantate von Hypophysenvorderlappen eine vorzeitige Ovarvergrößerung und Sexualreife bewirken (1926). In dem Interview, das *Michael Finkelstein* (F) 1966 mit *Bernhard Zondek* (Z) führte sagte *Zondek:* „We concluded that the pituitary and the placenta produce a hormonotrophin, a substance, which induced the ovaries to secrete the oestrogenic hormone. This was the first time, as far as I know, that a trophic hormone has been described". F: „Did you believe that the changes in the ovaries were induced by one pituitary hormone?" Z: „According to the histological changes of the ovaries we marked the reactions numerically from one to three. That is, we called the follicular maturation of the ovary under the influence of the pituitary ‚anterior pituitary reaction I', the appearance of ‚blood points" was called ‚APR II', and the formation of corpora lutea was termed ‚APR III'. Right from the

THE DISABILITIES CAUSED BY HYPO-
PHYSECTOMY AND THEIR
REPAIR

THE TUBERAL (HYPOTHALAMIC) SYNDROME
IN THE RAT *

PHILIP E. SMITH, PH.D.

Associate Professor of Anatomy, Stanford University School of Medicine

PALO ALTO, CALIF.

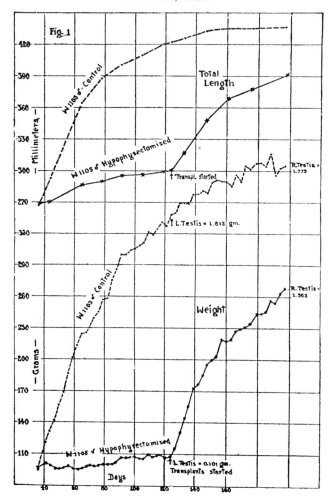

Growth rate of hypophysectomized rat before and after rat hypophysial transplants were given, and its control, not operated on: upper curve total length; lower curve, weight.

Smith, P. E.: The disabilities caused by hypophysectomy and their repair. J. Am. med. Ass. 88 (1927) 158–161 (Copyright 1921, American Medical Association).

beginning we believed that two pituitary hormones were essential for evoking these ovarian changes." Das Interview erfolgte anläßlich des 75. Geburtstags von *Zondek*. Die Publikation enthält das vollständige Literaturverzeichnis von *Zondeks* Arbeiten (*Zondek*, 1966).

Auf dem Kongreß der Deutschen Gesellschaft für Geburtshilfe und Gynäkologie am 22. Januar 1926 in Bonn und auf dem 1. Internationalen Kongreß für Sexualforschung im Oktober des gleichen Jahres in Berlin sagte *Zondek*: „Das Hypophysenvorderlappenhormon ist das übergeordnete, das allgemeine Sexualhormon. Der Hypophysenvorderlappen ist der Motor der Sexualfunktion. Durch unsere Implantationsversuche ist der exakte experimentelle Beweis geglückt, daß zwei endokrine Drüsen (Hypophysenvorderlappen und Ovarien) funktionelle Beziehungen haben, daß das Hormon einer endokrinen Drüse (Hypophysenvorderlappen) eine andere endokrine Drüse (Ovarium) zur Hormonproduktion anregt" (*Zondek* u. *Aschheim*, 1927). In der ausführlichen Publikation der Implantationsversuche wird als Datum der ersten Implantation der 8. Juli 1925 angegeben und gleichzeitig darauf hingewiesen, „*Smith* hat 10 Monate nach uns – im November 1926 – unabhängig von uns gleichartige Befunde wie wir am Ovarium der Ratte erhoben" (*Zondek* u. *Aschheim*, 1928). Anfangs vermuteten sie ein Hormon, später erkannten sie zwei Wirksubstanzen. Sie nannten diese Gonadotrophin oder Prolan A, das die Follikelreifung bewirkt und Prolan B, das die Ovulation auslöst und zur Corpus luteum-Bildung führt. Diese Annahme begründeten sie wie folgt: Reaktion I, Test für Prolan A: Follikelreifung, Ovulation, Follikelhormonbildung und Östrus; Reaktion II, Test für Prolan A und B: Hyperämie, Follikelhämatome (Blutpunkte); Reaktion III, Test für Prolan B: Luteinisierung und Bildung von Corpora lutea: Diese Befunde wurden in Frage gestellt (*J. B. Collip*, 1933, *E. C. Dodds*, 1934), bis zur Bestätigung durch die Untersuchungen von *Fevold, Hisaw* u. *Leonard* (1931) sowie *Hill* und *Parkes* (1931). Bereits 1930 schreibt *Zondek*: „Die weibliche Sexualfunktion spielt sich demnach in folgender Weise ab. Der Hypophysenvorderlappen ist der Motor der Sexualfunktion, das Hypophysenvorderlappenhormon, oder heute richtiger gesagt, die Hypophysenvorderlappenhormone sind die übergeordneten, allgemeinen, geschlechtsunspezifischen Sexualhormone. Das Prolan A löst die Follikelreifung aus, erzeugt in den follikulären Zellen (Thecazellen) das Folliculin, das seinerseits den Aufbau der Uterusschleimhaut bis zum Beginn der Sekretionsphase, d.h. der Proliferationsphase, auslöst. Das Prolan B bewirkt die Umwandlung der Granulosazellen in Luteinzellen und löst in den luteinisierten Granulosazellen den Cornerschen Stoff aus, den ich Lutin nennen möchte. Der Rhythmus im Hypophysenvor-

ÜBER DIE HORMONE DES HYPOPHYSENVORDER-LAPPENS.

I. Wachstumshormon, Follikelreifungshormon (Prolan A), Luteinisierungshormon (Prolan B), Stoffwechselhormon?

Von

Prof. Dr. BERNHARD ZONDEK.

Aus der geburtshilflich-gynäkologischen Abteilung des Städtischen Krankenhauses Berlin-Spandau (Prof. B. ZONDEK).

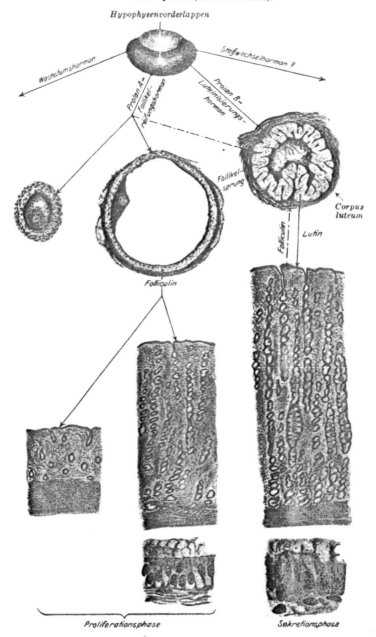

Abb. 1. Hypophysenvorderlappen und Genitalfunktion des Weibes.

Unsere bisherigen Arbeiten über das Hypophysenvorderlappenhormon (ZONDEK und ASCHHEIM[1]) müssen als bekannt vorausgesetzt werden. Wir konnten feststellen, daß das Hypophysenvorderlappenhormon das übergeordnete, das allgemeine, das geschlechtsunspezifische Sexualhormon ist. Am Ovarium des infantilen Nagetiers ruft die Implantation des Hypophysenvorderlappens eine Trias von morphologischen und funktionellen Reaktionen hervor, die wir folgendermaßen beschrieben:

HVR I = Follikelreifung, Ovulation, Auslösung des Folliculins im folliculären Apparat und dadurch sekundär Brunstreaktion;

HVR II = Massenblutung in erweiterte Follikel (= Blutpunkte);

HVR III = Luteinisierung (Bildung von echten Corpora lutea und Corpora lutea atretica).

◀ *Zondek*, B.: Über die Hormone des Hypophysenvorderlappens. Klin. Wochenschr. 9 (1930) 245–248 (© Springer Verlag).

derlappen in Quantität und Qualität, das rechtzeitige Einsetzen des Prolans B bedingt den Rhythmus der Ovarialfunktion, bedingt Proliferation und Funktion (Sekretion) der Uterusschleimhaut und schafft damit die optimalen Bedingungen für die Nidation des befruchteten Eis" (*Zondek*, 1930).

Philip E. Smith und seine Mitarbeiter beschrieben 1934, daß die Spermiogenese und die androgenetische Funktion der männlichen Keimdrüsen von verschiedenen gonadalen Stimuli abhängig sind (*Smith* u. *Leonhard*, 1934, *Smith* u. *Engle*, 1934, *Smith* et al., 1934). *Roy O. Greep* fand eine unterschiedliche Wirkung von FSH und LH bei hypophysektomierten unreifen und bei adulten Ratten. FSH hatte nur einen Effekt auf die Tubuli und LH stimulierte die Leydigzellen zur Androgensekretion (*Greep*, R. O. et al., 1936, *Greep* u. *Fevold*, 1937, *Greep*, 1937).

Choriongonadotropin

Eine endokrine Funktion der Plazenta wurde erstmals 1904 von *Josef Halban* an der I. Universitätsfrauenklinik in Wien bei *F. Schauta* postuliert. *Halban* untersuchte Organveränderungen bei weiblichen Früchten. „Ich hatte die Idee, ob nicht diese so wirksamen Substanzen, welche nach unserer heutigen Vorstellung im Blute der Mutter kreisen müssen, vielleicht auch durch die Plazenta in den fetalen Kreislauf gelangen und im fetalen Organismus ähnliche Reaktionen wie bei der Mutter hervorrufen." Er fand schwangerschaftsbedingte Veränderungen am Uterus, den Mammae und der Prostata, die sich nach der Geburt wieder zurückbilden. „Ich selbst habe schon die Vermutung ausgesprochen, daß es sich hierbei um eine Wirkung der Plazenta handle und daß es mir als wahrscheinlich vorkommt, daß speziell das Chorionepithel durch innere Sekretion Substanzen abscheide, welche, einerseits in den mütterlichen, andererseits in den fetalen Kreislauf aufgenommen, in beiden Organismen analoge Reaktionen hervorbringen." Auch bei der Blasenmole und „Missed labour" fanden sich die gleichen Veränderungen, wor-

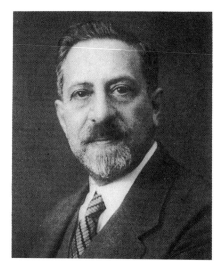

Halban, J. (1870–1937 in Wien): Assistent bei Schauta, Pionier der Endokrinologie der Reproduktion.

aus er schloß, daß diese nicht vom lebenden Fetus ausgehen können (*Halban*, 1904). Ein Jahr später untermauerte *Halban* seine Vorstellungen in einer 88 Seiten umfassenden Arbeit mit 145 Literaturzitaten im Archiv für Gynäkologie: „Die innere Sekretion von Ovarien und Plazenta und ihre Bedeutung für die Funktion der Milchdrüse" (*Halban* 1905). Hier stellte er jeweils nach Erörterung von klinischen Beobachtungen folgende Thesen auf:

„I. Der Pubertätsimpuls der Mammae des normalen Weibes ist von Stoffen abhängig, welche vom Ovarium abgesondert werden.

II. Die menstruellen Veränderungen der Mamma sind von chemischen Stoffen abhängig, welche vom Ovarium stammen.

III. Die Ovarien stellen in der Schwangerschaft nicht, wie dies außerhalb derselben der Fall, das trophische Zentrum des übrigen Genitales und der Mamma dar. Ihre Funktion ist in dieser Hinsicht während der Schwangerschaft nicht von Bedeutung.

IV. Auf die Schwangerschaftshyperplasie der Mamma und auf die Milchsekretion haben die Ovarien keinen Einfluß.

VI. Die Schwangerschaftsveränderungen der Mammae können nicht von den Stoffwechselprodukten der Frucht ausgelöst werden, da sie auch trotz längeren Abgestorbenseins der Frucht erhalten bleiben.

VII. Der Fruchtkörper kann überhaupt nichts mit der Auslösung der Schwangerschaftsreaktion zu tun haben.

VIII. Die aktiven Schwangerschaftssubstanzen sind ein Effekt der Plazenta bzw. des Trophoblastes und Chorionepithel.

IX. Der erste oder embryonale Wachstumsimpuls der Mamma ist als ein Effekt der Plazentarsubstanzen aufzufassen.

X. ... daß wir es hier mit einer ganz allgemeinen Eigenschaft der Plazentar- und Ovarialstoffe zu tun haben, Hyperämie und Hämorrhagien zu erzeugen.

XI. ... daß von den ovariellen und plazentaren Substanzen ganz analoge Wirkungen ausgeübt werden, nur daß der Effekt der plazentaren Stoffe ein wesentlich intensiverer ist.

XII. Während der Gravidität übernimmt die Plazenta die protektive Funktion des Ovarium und führt sie potenziert durch.

XIII. ... daß dem Uterus weder bei der Geburt noch im Puerperium eine Bedeutung in dieser Frage zukommt, denn wir sehen, daß die Milchsekretion sich stets in ganz gleicher Weise einstellt, mag nun der Uterus vorhanden sein oder nicht.

Z. Geburtsh. u. Gynäkol. 53, 191–231, 1904

VIII.

Schwangerschaftsreaktionen der fötalen Organe und ihre puerperale Involution.

Von

Privatdozent Dr. Josef Halban.

Die auffallenden und mannigfachen Veränderungen des mütterlichen Organismus in der Schwangerschaft werden in neuerer Zeit wohl mit Recht als der Effekt von chemischen Substanzen angesehen, welche in der Schwangerschaft erzeugt werden und im Blute der Mutter zirkulieren. Diese Reaktionen betreffen vor allem den Genitalapparat und die Brustdrüsen, in welchen Veränderungen gesetzt werden, die für die Entwicklung der Frucht im intrauterinen und postembryonalen Leben von höchster Bedeutung sind.

Daß es sich bei den Schwangerschaftsveränderungen in der Mamma tatsächlich um chemische Wirkungen handelt, dafür sprechen die bekannten Versuche von Goltz [1] und Ribbert [2].

Daß aber auch für die Schwangerschaftsveränderungen des Uterus (Hyperämie, Hypertrophie, Deciduabildung) ein ähnliches chemisches Prinzip existieren muß, dafür sprechen die Beobachtungen an Extrauteringraviditäten. Bei diesen kommt es zu denselben Reaktionen des Uterus, wie bei normalem Sitze des Eies, was wohl bei der Fernwirkung nur auf chemische Reize zurückgeführt werden kann.

Neben den zweckmäßigen Reaktionen im Genitale und in der Mamma gibt es noch eine Reihe anderer Veränderungen, welche während der Schwangerschaft im mütterlichen Organismus auftreten, deren Zweckmäßigkeit nicht ohne weiteres einzusehen ist, die aber doch in Analogie mit den ersteren als chemische Reaktionen auf aktive Substanzen aufgefaßt werden müssen, z. B. die Pigmentation der Haut, die Bildung der Varikositäten an den Extremitäten, Veränderungen in der Blutbeschaffenheit, psychische Veränderungen etc.

Ich hatte nun die Idee, ob nicht diese so wirksamen Substanzen, welche nach unserer heutigen Vorstellung im Blute der Mutter kreisen müssen, vielleicht auch durch die Placenta in den fötalen Kreislauf gelangen und im fötalen Organismus ähnliche Reaktionen wie bei der Mutter hervorrufen.

Schlußsätze.

1. Wir haben Gründe anzunehmen, daß die Schwangerschafts-reaktionen des mütterlichen Organismus auf die Wirkung chemischer Stoffe zurückzuführen sind.

2. Bei der Frucht finden sich ganz ähnliche Veränderungen, wie bei der Mutter.

3. Der weibliche Fötus weist, ebenso wie die Mutter, eine Schwangerschaftshypertrophie und Hyperämie der Gebärmutter auf.

4. Die deziduale Reaktion der mütterlichen Gebärmutter scheint beim Fötus ihre Analogie in einer menstruellen Reaktion zu haben.

5. Die bekannten Genitalblutungen neugeborener Mädchen sind der höchste Grad dieser Reaktion.

6. Die Mamma des Fötus hypertrophiert während der Schwanger-schaft ganz ähnlich wie die mütterliche und zeigt eigentümliche histologische Veränderungen.

7. Ebenso reagiert bei männlichen Früchten die Mamma und die Prostata mit Hypertrophie und denselben eigentümlichen histologi-schen Veränderungen wie die Mamma weiblicher Früchte.

8. Ebenso ist beim Fötus die Wirkung der Schwangerschafts-gifte eine analoge wie bei der Mutter (Leukozytose, Fibrinvermeh-rung, Nierenschädigung, Oedeme).

9. Wir haben Gründe, um anzunehmen, daß die aktiven Schwangerschaftssubstanzen von der Placenta stammen, deren Chorion-epithel eine innere Sekretion zugesprochen werden muß.

10. Nach der Geburt fallen die von der Placenta abgeschiedenen Substanzen fort und es kommt sowohl bei der Mutter als beim Kind zu einer puerperalen Involution aller Organe, welche während der Gravidität hypertrophierten und zur Regeneration aller durch die Giftwirkung geschädigten Organe.

11. Die Eklampsie ist der Effekt einer stärkeren Giftwirkung der schon bei normaler Schwangerschaft auftretenden Gifte.

Die Eklampsiegifte stammen dementsprechend ebenfalls von der Placenta, zirkulieren im mütterlichen und fötalen Organismus und erzeugen bei beiden die analogen Veränderungen.

Halban, J.: Schwangerschaftsreaktionen der fötalen Organe und ihre puerperale Involution. (Mit Genehmigung F. Enke-Verlag). Z. Geburts. Gynäkol. 53 (1904) 191–231

XIV. Die Auslösung der Milchsekretion kann nicht durch nervöse Impulse ausgelöst werden.

XV. Die Milchabsonderung wird nicht durch den Saugakt ausgelöst. Dieser wirkt nur befördernd auf eine bereits bestehende Sekretion ein und unterhält diese.

XV. ... gegen die Hypothese zu sprechen, daß die durch die Geburt veränderten Zirkulationsverhältnisse und eine dadurch entstehende Hyperämie zu der Mamma die milchauslösende Ursache darstellt.

XVI. ... daß der Geburtstakt als solcher nicht als die Ursache für das Auftreten der Milchsekretion anzusehen ist.

XVII. Die puerperale Involution ist nichts anderes, als eine echte Atrophie, welche physiologischer Weise durch die Ausschaltung der Plazenta hervorgerufen wird.

XVIII. ... es nicht der Wegfall des Fruchtkörpers sein kann, welcher die Milchsekretion auslöst.

XIX. ... so zeigen die eben beschriebenen Fälle von Blasenmole, daß es nur die Plazenta bzw. das Chorionepithel sein kann, deren biologische Ausschaltung den Anstoß zur Milchsekretion gibt.

XX. Das Ovarium wirkt in geeigneten Fällen ganz ähnlich – nur in der Regel quantitativ schwächer – wie die Plazenta und zwar nicht nur hyperplasierend auf das Mammagewebe, sondern auch hemmend auf dessen Sekretion.

XXI. Milchsekretion bei männlichen Individuen dürfte dadurch zu Stande kommen, daß bei Gynäkomastien die Wirkung der Testikel in Wegfall kommt."

Halban begründet seine Thesen allein auf klinischen Beobachtungen, als Versuche, die die Natur selbst vorgenommen hat. Der Biologe *James T. Bradbury* in Iowa City weist 1955 auf die Bedeutung der Halban'schen Arbeit hin. „His concept is based on deductive reasoning made possible by astute clinical observations. His presentation is an outstanding example of how careful observation and evaluation can produce a true concept when each case is clearly valid evidence and there is no need for statistical consideration" (*Bradbury*, 1955). H. H. *Simmer* hat *Halbans* Arbeiten sorgfältig analysiert und eingeordnet (*Simmer*, 1984, 1985).

Otfried O. Fellner (1873– ~ 1936) am Institut für allgemeine und experimentelle Pathologie in Wien bei *R. Paltauf* äußerte sich kritisch zu *Halbans* Thesen und erbrachte selbst den experimentellen Beweis für die endokrine Funktion der Plazenta (*Fellner*, 1913). Mit Plazentaextrakten erzielte

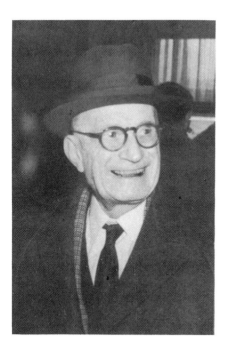

S. Aschheim (1878–1965): Gynäkologe in Berlin, 1936 Emigration nach Paris. Testverfahren an der infantilen Maus zum Gonadotropinnachweis. Aschheim-Zondek-Schwangerschaftstest (siehe Zondek) (1960).

er Genitalveränderungen auch ohne Vermittlung der Ovarien, d.h. bei kastrierten Tieren. „In der Plazenta, den Eihäuten, den Corpus luteum-haltigen Ovarien sind Stoffe enthalten, welche bei subkutaner und intraperitonealer Injektion Wachstum der Mamma und Mamilla, Vergrößerung des Uterus, Brunst- bzw. Graviditätserscheinungen an der Schleimhaut des Uterus, Vergrößerung der Graviditätserscheinungen an der Vagina, parenchymatöse Nephritis und Ausbleiben des Wachstums ausrasierter Haare hervorrufen."

F. Binz erzielte mit Serum gravider Frauen bei infantilen Mäusen eine Vergrößerung des Uterus. „Er weist auf die Möglichkeit der Schwangerschaftsdiagnostik mit dieser Methode hin, und es entbehrt nicht einer gewissen Tragik, wenn er schreibt, daß er aus ‚äußerlichen Gründen' diese Arbeit nicht fortführen kann, daß er sie aber für aussichtsreich hält" (*Binz*, 1924, zit. nach *Blobel*, 1966).

Als Histologe kannte *Aschheim* die Veränderungen der Hypophyse in der Schwangerschaft und schloß daraus auf eine gesteigerte Funktion. *Erdheim* und *Stumma* (1909) hatten typische Veränderungen der Hypophyse in der Schwangerschaft beschrieben. Auf dem Gynäkologenkongreß in Bonn 1927 berichtete *Aschheim* über gonadotrope Aktivität sowohl in der Plazenta, als

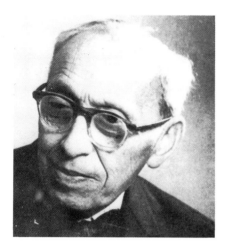

Zondek, B. (1891–1966): Gynäkologe in Berlin; 1934 Emigration nach Jerusalem. 1926 zus. mit Aschheim die Entdeckung der Wirkung von Hypophysenimplantaten auf das Ovar, 1927 Gonadotropingehalt in Schwangeren-Urin, 1930 zwei gonadotrope Faktoren im Urin postmenopausaler Frauen.

auch im Schwangeren Urin. *Aschheim* und *Zondek* an der Charité in Berlin nahmen fälschlicherweise an, daß das Hormon aus der Hypophyse stammt. Ihre Untersuchungen führten zur Entwicklung eines Schwangerschaft-Tests mit infantilen Mäusen. Der Test diente über mehr als 30 Jahre als zuverlässiger und allgemein benutztes Verfahren zum Nachweis einer Gravidität.

Selmar Aschheim (˙ 1878 Berlin – † 1965 Paris) arbeitete von 1912 bis 1935 in der Frauenklinik der Charité in Berlin. Er mußte Deutschland 1936 verlassen und ging nach Paris, wo er am Centre National de la Recherche Scientifique arbeitete. *Bernhard Zondek* (˙ 1891 Wronke – 1966 New York) kam 1919 an die Charité. 1929 wurde er Leiter der Frauenabteilung in Berlin-Spandau. Schon 1933 mußte er Deutschland verlassen. Nach einer kurzen Zeit in Stockholm bei *Hans Euler* übersiedelte er nach Israel und im Alter von 75 Jahren an das Albert Einstein College in New York.

Immer wieder gibt es Hinweise in der Literatur, daß die alten Ägypter schon durch Untersuchungen des Harns versucht haben sollen, eine Schwangerschaft zu diagnostizieren. Die unterschiedliche Keimung von Getreidekörnern wurde hierzu herangezogen. *Blobel* (1966) zeigte, daß hCG das Wachstum von Weizenkeimlingen hemmt.

Murata und *Adachi* (1927) konnten durch Verabreichung von Blasenmolengewebe, Chorionepitheliom und Plazenta bei Kaninchen Corpora lutea induzieren. Sie postulierten, daß die wirksame Substanz aus den Zottenepithelien der Plazenta stammt und die Aufgabe habe, das Corpus luteum graviditatis zu schützen. Die Autoren zitieren eine Arbeit von *Hirose* von

menschlichem Hypophysenvorderlappen, wobei es ebenso wie beim Tier gleichgültig ist, ob die Hypophyse von einem männlichen oder weiblichen Organismus stammt. Wir begnügen uns

4. Das Hypophysenvorderlappenhormon ist bei Mensch und Tier identisch. Das Hormon findet sich in der Hypophyse des männlichen und weiblichen Organismus.

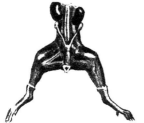
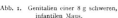

Abb. 1. Genitalien einer 8 g schweren, infantilen Maus.

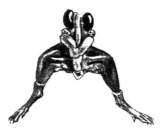

Abb. 2. Genitalien einer 8 g schweren, infantilen, durch Hypophysenvorderlappen in sexuelle Frühreife gebrachten Maus.

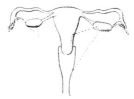

Abb. 3. Wirkung des im Ovarium gebildeten Ovarialhormons auf das Erfolgsorgan.

hier mit der kurzen Wiedergabe unserer Resultate, die ausführliche Mitteilung und Literaturangabe erfolgt im Archiv für Gynäkologie.

Unsere Versuche ergeben:

1. Die Ovarialfunktion kann auf unspezifische Weise nicht angeregt werden.

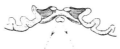

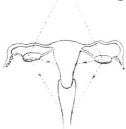

Abb. 4. Wirkung des dem Körper zugeführten Ovarialhormons (Folliculin) auf das Erfolgsorgan (Uterus, Scheide) und auf das Ovarium.

Abb. 5. Wirkung des Hypophysenvorderlappenhormons auf das Ovarium. Das im Ovarium mobilisierte Ovarialhormon wirkt auf sein Erfolgsorgan (Uterus, Scheide).

5. *Das Hypophysenvorderlappenhormon ist das übergeordnete, das allgemeine Sexualhormon. Der Hypophysenvorderlappen ist der Motor der Sexualfunktion.*

Durch unsere Implantationsversuche ist der exakte experimentelle Beweis geglückt, daß zwei endokrine Drüsen (Hypophysenvorderlappen und Ovarium) funktionelle Beziehungen haben, daß das Hormon einer endokrinen Drüse (Hypophysenvorderlappen) eine andere endokrine Drüse (Ovarium) zur Hormonproduktion anregt.

DAS HORMON DES HYPOPHYSENVORDER-LAPPENS[*]).

I. Testobjekt zum Nachweis des Hormons.

Von

Prof. Dr. BERNHARD ZONDEK und Dr. S. ASCHHEIM.

Aus der Universitäts-Frauenklinik der Charité zu Berlin
(Direktor: Geh. Med.-Rat Prof. Dr. K FRANZ †).

[*] Nach einem Vortrag, gehalten in der Berliner Gesellschaft für Geburtshilfe und Gynäkologie am 22. Januar 1926 und auf dem I. internationalen Kongreß für Sexualforschung in Berlin (Oktober 1926).

Zondek, B., S. Aschheim: Das Hormon des Hypophysenvorderlappens. Klin. Wochenschr. 6 (1927) 247–252 (© Springer-Verlag).

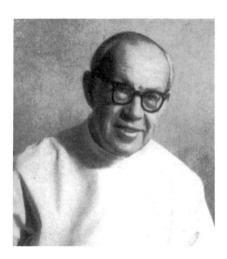

Philipp, E. (1893–1961): Ass. bei Ernst Bumm und Walter Stoeckel an der Charité Frauenklinik in Berlin, 1934 Greifswald, 1937 Kiel. 1930 Nachweis von gonadotroper Aktivität in der Plazenta.

1920, der in der Vermehrung der Langhans-Zellen zu Anfang der Gravidität den Ausdruck einer gesteigerten innersekretorischen Aktivität sah.

Der Nachweis des extrahypophysären Ursprungs des hCG nämlich die Plazenta erfolgte 1930 durch *E. Philipp* und gleichzeitig durch *J. B. Collip.* *Ernst Philipp* (1893–1961) in der Frauenklinik bei Stöckel in Berlin zeigte, daß Hypophysenimplantate von Schwangeren bei immaturen Mäusen keine Reaktion bewirkten, dagegen Plazentastücke eine weit stärkere Ovarreaktion induzierten, vor allem auch Choriongewebe aus hydatiformen Molen und Chorionepitheliom. „Die Plazenta tritt also in der Gravidität in den Kreis der innersekretorischen Drüsen ein und stimmt sie in typischer Weise um. Wie sie mit dem Ovar und dem Corpus luteum in wechselseitige Beziehung tritt, geschieht dies auch mit dem Hypophysenvorderlappen. Neben dem brunstauslösenden Stoff produziert sie das, den positiven Ausfall der Aschheim-Zondekschen Schwangerschaftsreaktion bedingende, „Vorderlappenhormon". Dies letztere ist für den Hypophysenvorderlappen ebensowenig spezifisch wie das weibliche Sexualhormon für den Eierstock" (*Philipp*, 1930).

James B. Collip (1892–1965) an der McGill University in Toronto vermutete in einer preliminary communication im Canadian Medical Journal „that the placenta may produce an ovarian stimulating hormone" (Collip, 1930). *Vozza* konnte nie in Hypophysen von Schwangeren, aber im Plazentagewebe gonadotrope Aktivitäten nachweisen (*Vozza*, 1932). *I. Kido* an der Frauenklinik der kaiserlichen Kyushu-Universität in Fukuoka, Japan, transplantierte Plazentagewebe in die Augenvorderkammer des Kaninchen. Im Gegensatz zu intramuskulären Transplantaten, fand im Auge ein Verwachsen

Zentralblatt für Gynäkologie 1930. Nr. 8.

Aus d. Univ.-Frauenklinik Berlin.   Direktor: Geh.-Rat Prof. W. Stoeckel.

Hypophysenvorderlappen und Placenta.

Von Priv.-Doz. Dr. E. Philipp, Assistent der Klinik.

Im Zbl. Gynäk. 1929, Nr 38 konnte ich zeigen, daß die Placenta verschiedener Tiere nicht Speicherungs-, sondern Bildungsstätte des brunstauslösenden Stoffes (Follikulin, Oestrin usw.) ist. Dasselbe gilt von der menschlichen Placenta, wie Waldstein und Verf. nachgewiesen haben. Ich sprach weiter auf Grund meiner Untersuchungen bei Blasenmole die Behauptung aus, daß auch das »Vorderlappenhormon« in der Gravidität von der Placenta gebildet wird, und daß die Schwangerschaftsreaktion von Aschheim und Zondek in Wirklichkeit eine Placenta-

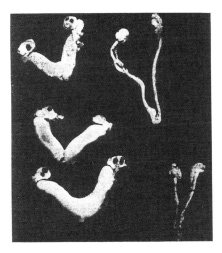

Philipp, E.: Hypophysenvorderlappen und Placenta. Zentralbl. Gyn. 39 (1930) 450– 453.

Fig. 1.
Links die Genitalorgane von 3 infantilen Mäusen, denen die Chorionzotten einer Grav. mens. II implantiert wurden. Rechts 2 Kontrollen. (Versuch 44.)

Am. J. Obstet. Gyn. 61, 1951, 990–1000

HORMONE SECRETION BY HUMAN PLACENTA GROWN IN THE EYES OF RABBITS*†

H. L. Stewart, Jr., M.D., Detroit, Mich.

(From the Department of Obstetrics and Gynecology and The Edsel B. Ford Institute for Medical Research, Henry Ford Hospital)

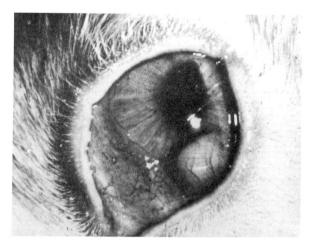

Fig. 3.—Photograph of the eye of Rabbit No. 2 at the end of the eighteenth week. The placental tissue has grown from a small implant measuring 0.5 mm. to a large, well-vascularized growth.

mit dem Irisgewebe statt, es fanden sich Mitosen der Langhans'schen Zellen und eine Sprossung des Synzytium. In den Ovarien der Tiere zeigte sich eine Follikelreifung und der Harn eine positive Aschheim-Zondek'sche Reaktion. „Damit habe ich meines Erachtens experimentell sicher nachgewiesen, daß die menschlichen Chorionepithelien das die Aschheim-Zondeck'sche Schwangerschaftsreaktion hervorrufende Hormon produzieren" (*Kido*, 1937). *Gey* und Mitarbeiter demonstrierten die Produktion von hCG durch Trophoblastzellen in Kultur (*Gey* et al., 1938). Von der Arbeitsgruppe von *A. Westman* am Karolinska Institut in Stockholm wurde 1948 über kristallines hCG und dessen biologische Wirkung berichtet (*Claesson* et al., 1948). *H. L. Stewart* vom Henry Ford Hospital in Detroit kritisierte in einem Vortrag 1950 die Versuche von *Kido*, weil in diesen die Transplantatwirkung nur

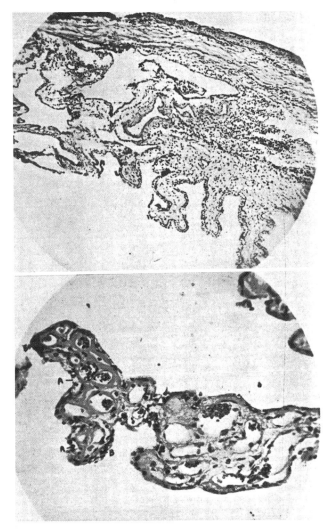

Fig. 4.—Photomicrographs showing growth of placental villi in the rabbit's eye (upper). (×50.) Higher power (lower) demonstrates Langhans cells (A) and collections of syncytial cells (B). (×430.)

Stewart, H. I.: Hormone secretion by human placenta grown in the eyes of rabbits. Am. J. Obstet. Gyn. 61 (1951) 990–1000 (permission Mosby Year Book Inc., St. Louis). Read at the 18 annual meeting of the central Association of Obstetricians and Gynecologists, Milwaukee, Wis. Sept. (1950).

THE POTENCY OF BLOOD SERUM OF MARES IN PROGRESSIVE STAGES OF PREGNANCY IN EFFECTING THE SEXUAL MATURITY OF THE IMMATURE RAT

H. H. COLE AND G. H. HART

From the College of Agriculture, University of California, Davis

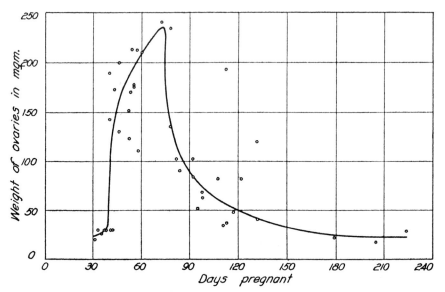

Fig. 1. Graph shows average weights of ovaries of rats injected with serum taken from mares at various stages of pregnancy. Weights include ovaries with oviducts and bursae attached.

Cole, H. H., G. H. Hart: The potency of blood serum of mares in progressive stages of pregnancy in effecting the sexual maturity of the immature rat. Am. J. Physiol. 93 (1930) 57–68 (Permission granted by The American Physiol. Society).

auf einen Zeitraum bis zu 18 Tagen verfolgt wurde (*Stewart*, 1951). „My study shows that absorption of gonadotropin present in the decidua of human pregnancy will give a positive gonadotropin response in the ovaries of rabbits, but as the explant continues to grow additional evidence of the decidual tissue as the site of formation of the hormone is lacking. It is believed from this study with growth of the placental cells over a period of four to six months that the placenta is the site of formation of estrogens and gonadotropin" (*Stewart*, 1951).

Die Promotionsarbeit von *Egon Diczfalusy* von 1953 hat den Titel „Chorionic gonadotropin and estrogens in the human placenta". Die Frage nach der Herkunft von hCG war nun endgültig geklärt und es begann die Untersuchung der Physiologie der Plazenta. Es wurde das Konzept der Fetoplazentaren Einheit entwickelt (*Diczfalusy* 1953, 1960).

1930 wurde gonadotrope Aktivität auch im Serum trächtiger Stuten gefunden; PMSG, pregnant mare serum gonadotropin (*H. H. Cole* u. *G. H. Hart* 1930, *Zondek* 1930). „The blood of 62 mares was tested for its potency in inducing the sexual maturity of immature rats. Serum from non-pregnant mares was negative in all instances as was the serum of mares up to the 37th day of pregnancy. The time of pregnancy at which the serum first gave a positive reaction varied in different individuals from the 37th to the 42nd day" (*Cole* and *Hart,* 1930). PMSG wird in den endometrial cups und nicht in der Plazenta produziert.

HCG-ähnliche Aktivität wurde bei Primaten nachgewiesen. *Van Wagenen* und *Simpson* bestimmten die Gonadotropinausscheidung bei schwangeren Affen biologisch und immunologisch (1955, 1970). Im biologischen Test mit hypophysektomierten Ratten fanden sich zwischen Tag 22 und 34 positive Werte, mit immunologischen hCG-Tests zwischen Tag 20 und 30 positive Befunde.

Follikelstimulierendes und Luteinisierendes Hormon

Der Chemiker *Harry L. Fevold* und der Biologe *Frederick L. Hisaw* (· 1891 Jolly/Missouri – † 1972 Cambridge/Mass.) am Department of Zoology, University of Wisconsin erbrachten den Nachweis daß Follikelwachstum und die nachfolgende Luteinisierung durch zwei voneinander zu unterscheidende Faktoren, die sie gonad stimulating und luteinizing hormone nannten, kontrolliert werden.

1. „The anterior lobe of the hypophysis secretes two hormones which act on the ovary, a gonad stimulating factor which stimulates follicular growth and a luteinizing factor which causes lutein growth.
2. These two hormones have been extracted, quantitatively from dried anterior lobe tissue by means of aqueous pyridine.
3. The two hormones have been separated from another into two different preparations each of which gives a different physiological reaction. When the two fractions are again united the resulting preparation is entirely similar to the first crude extract.
4. The luteinizing hormone cannot act on the immature ovary. The infantile ovary must be stimulated to follicular activity by the gonad stimulating hormone before a characteristic ‚mulberry' ovary can be produced" (*Fevold* et al., 1931).

Die Befunde bestätigten sich mit weiter gereinigten Präparaten (*Fevold* u. *Hisaw,* 1934): „The FSH and LH act together on the ovary to produce macroscopic follicles and corpora lutea. Both seem to have separate functions to perform in 1, 2, 3, 4 sequence which must take place in the order designated. Each hormone is dependent on the previous action of the other on the ovary and consequently the combined effects of the two on the ovaries of rats as measured by the weight and appearance of the ovaries are greater than would be expected from the results obtained by injecting each separately in different animals. The effect of each hormone has been augmented by the action of each other."

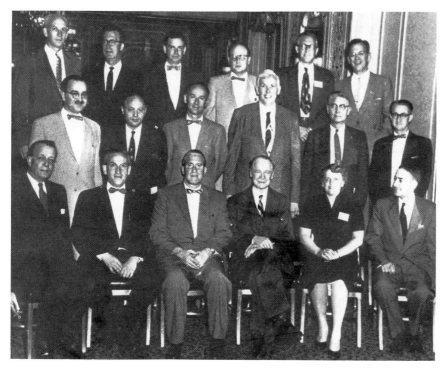

Arbeitsgruppe F. L. Hisaw, 1956 (Genehmigung R. O. Greep) (1. Reihe von li.: Ch. Hamre, R. Hertz, R. K. Meyer, F. L. Hisaw, V. Mayo Fiske, E. B. Astwood. – 2. Reihe: M. X. Zarrow, A. Albert, M. A. Foster, R. J. Bailey, W. H. Schaefer, A. A. Hellbaum. – 3. Reihe: R. O. Greep, C. A. Bunde, C. T. G. King, H. A. Salhanick, R. V. Talmage, R. L. Kroc).

Roy Orvall Greep (˙1905 Longford, Kansas), der 1930 zu *Hisaw* ging, beschreibt die mühsamen Experimente eindrucksvoll in seiner Dale-Lecture 1967. „*Fevold,* the chemist, and *Hisaw,* the biologist, were engaged in an effort to extract the gonad-stimulating activities of the pituitary. They had taken the position that the growth of ovarian follicles and their subsequent luteinization were controlled by different physiological principles which they had already come to refer as FSH and LH. But the implied hormonal status was a fair distance ahead of the available facts. The problem was to separate these two activities. Since the luteinizing factor seemed susceptile to destruction at acid pH and the yield of FSH was poor at alkaline pH an amphoteric solution of aqueous pyridine was used as the extraction medium of choice. I hardly need mention that the yield was satisfactory but it was also a fact that the laboratory was not equipped with ventilating hoods. The weekly routine at the closing hour on friday was to place a pan containing a litre of 30 % py-

THE GONAD STIMULATING AND THE LUTEINIZING HORMONES OF THE ANTERIOR LOBE OF THE HYPOPHESIS[1]

H. L. FEVOLD, F. L. HISAW AND S. L. LEONARD

From the Department of Zoology, University of Wisconsin

Received for publication February 16, 1931

The existence of a relationship between the anterior lobe of the pituitary gland and the ovaries of vertebrate animals has been definitely established. Facts which support this relationship are so well known that it is not deemed necessary to give a comprehensive review of the literature, since it may be found elsewhere (Fluhmann, 1929).

The evidence for the secretion of two distinct hormones by the anterior lobe of the hypophysis, namely, a growth hormone and a hormone functioning as a gonad stimulator, seems to be rather definite. On the other hand, while various authors have put forth the idea that there are two different hormones secreted by this gland, which act on the ovary, still no very definite evidence is at hand proving this contention. Zondek (1930a, b) gives indirect evidence of this idea, since his preparations from urine give two different pictures in the ovaries of rats, depending on the source of the urine. Evans and Simpson (1928) believe that there are two substances present which affect the ovary, but that one, namely, the luteinizing hormone is identical with the growth hormone. Claus (1931) offers good experimental evidence for the presence of two different substances in the anterior lobe which act on the ovary. However, as will be shown later, the substances which she obtained do not seem to be the same as those with which we are dealing.

In this paper we wish to present definite evidence for the presence of two distinct anterior lobe hormones which promote follicular and lutein development in the ovary. One of these is the gonad stimulating hormone

TABLE 4

Effect of gonad stimulating, luteinizing hormone and combination of the two on the ovaries of immature rats. Equivalent of 0.02 gram dried anterior lobe powder injected daily for 5 days

RAT NUMBER	VAGINA AT AUTOPSY	SMEAR	OVARIES	WEIGHT OF OVARIES		PER CENT INCREASE
				Experimental	Control	
				mgm.	*mgm.*	
1234	Open	Oestrous	Follicles	21.2	9.8	116
1246	Open	Oestrous	Follicles	28.5	10.4	174
1232	Open	Oestrous	Follicles	31.6	9.8	212
1233	Open	Oestrous	Follicles	22.7	9.8	131
1225	Closed		Infantile	13.6	12.1	
1230	Closed		Infantile	16.3	14.3	
1228	Closed		Infantile	12.2	13.2	
1229	Closed		Infantile	13.5	13.2	
1238	Open	Leucocytes	C.L. and F.	117.5	10.7	996
1240	Open	Leucocytes	C.L. and F.	83.0	9.4	771
1241	Open	Leucocytes	C.L. and F.	104.0	9.8	963

Fevold, H. L., F. L. Hisaw, S. L. Leonard: The gonad stimulating and the luteinizing hormones of the anterior lobe of the hypophesis. Am. J. Physiol. 97 (1931) 291–301 (permission granted The American Physiologic Soc.).

ridine and a few grammes of precious sheep pituitary powder before an electric fan in the open. On Monday morning the parched residue, greenish in colour and criss-crossed with cracks was ready for extraction. What happened over the weekend is worthy of recording. The extraction procedure was carried out on the upper floor. Within minutes the vaporous fumes of pyridine, nearing the lethal level in the laboratory, would start seeping beneath the door and into the hallway. The downward migration of these fumes was halted only by the lower-most of the subterranean reaches of the building. Anyone familiar with the smell of pyridine at nausceous level will appreciate that the Friday evening exodus of invertebrate zoologists, cytologists, embryologists and botanists from that building was not entirely voluntary. No one complained. It was all in the interest of science, and research on sex matters was somewhat adventurous in those days. To those of us in endocrinology the smell of pyridine meant hormones for our studies and we carried on as usual. Why we did not all lose our livers remains a pharmacological mystery. – The question whether hypophysial ovarian control involved one or two gonadotrophic hormones became a matter of sharp division of opinion. The difficulty, as everyone knew, was that the purification and separation procedures and the biological assay were crude and inadequate. It was clearly possible to prepare a follicle-stimulating extract that would incite pure follicle development in immature rats over a four day period. But, if the dose were raised sufficiently or the period of treatment was extended to five days corpora lutea would appear. The evidence was admittedly damaging but it was argued that the luteinization was due to LH originating from the test animal's own pituitary. The one-hormone school held that luteinization was an intrinsic property of, and natural sequence in the growth and development of an ovarian follicle. ... More and more it came to be appreciated that the matter could not be settled without the use of hypophysectomized rats. If *Smith* at Columbia hadn't already performed that operation, one would have been quick to conclude from the anatomical situation alone that it was a surgical impossibility. *Smith's* published description of the operative procedure was sparing of details and not designed to spawn a generation of rat-pituitary surgeons." *Greep* schildert dann den mühsamen Weg bis es gelang, hypophysektomierte Tiere zu bekommen und die FSH- und LH-Fraktionen in diesen zu testen. „The outcome left virtually nothing to be desired. The FSH ovaries were greatly enlarged and by transmitted light showed no telltale signs of luteinization. The ovaries and uteri of LH treated rats were not distinguishable from those of the operated controls. This was the end of an era of gnawing uncertainty. We had not solved the problem but the outcome

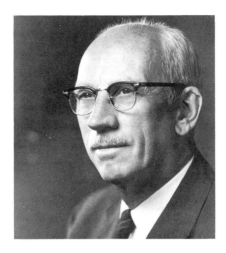

Greep, R. O. 1905: Assistent bei Hisaw, 1938 Squibb Institute for medical Research in Brusnwick mit Harry van Dyke und Bacon Chow; 1944 Harvard. Bei Hisaw Nachweis von FSH und LH-Aktivität; Prostatalappentest mit van Dyke und Chow; Wachstumshormonwirkung; 1953 Greep's Histology; 1969 Reproduction and Human Wefare: A Challenge to Research, Frontiers in Reproduction and Fertility Control.

was no longer in doubt. It was the beginning of an era in which headway could be made toward the chemical purification and isolation of these biological entities through the use of valid biological indicators" (*Greep*, 1967).

Carl Kaufmann (1900–1980) erzielte durch alleinige Verabreichung großer Östrogendosen bei drei Frauen mit sekundärer Amenorrhö eine sekretorische Umwandlung des Endometriums und echte Menstruation. *Kaufmann* spricht von der Notwendigkeit eines Östrogenanstiegs für die Ausschüttung von Gonadotropinen. „In diesen Fällen muß der eigene Gehalt des Ovars an Follikelhormon nicht ausgereicht haben, um auf dem Umwege über die Hypophyse die Luteinisierung des Follikels und hierdurch die Schleimhautfunktion und Menstruation zu erregen" (*Kaufmann*, 1933). *Hohlweg* bestätigte die von *Kaufmann* bei der Frau gefundene positive Rückkopplung bei Ratten (*Hohlweg*, 1934). Eine zusammenfassende Besprechung der Befunde zur Zyklusregulation findet man in der Monographie von *C. Clauberg* von 1933: „Die weiblichen Sexualhormone, in ihren Beziehungen zum Genitalzyklus und zum Hypophysenvorderlappen".

Roy Hertz (⁕ 1909 Cleveland) behandelte in seiner Doktorarbeit 1934 die ovulationsauslösende Wirkung von Gonadotropinen bei juvenilen Kaninchen. „The occurrence of ovulation only after a combined treatment with FSH and LH throws some light upon the physiology of ovulation, indicating that this process may depend on a synergistic balance between the two gonadotropic hormones" (*Hertz* u. *Hisaw*, 1934).

H. M. Evans publizierte 1936 Befunde, die ICSH als ein von LH und von FSH zu unterscheidendes Hormon beweisen sollten. *Fevold* wiederholte

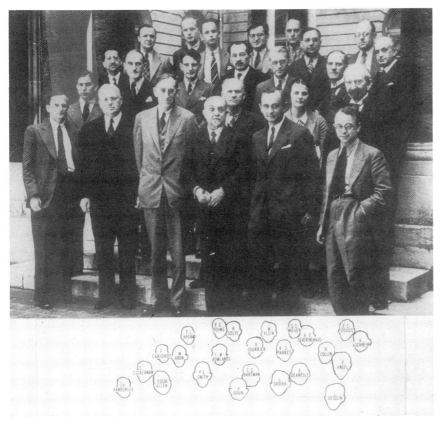

Early pioneers in anterior pituitary physiology, Singer Poliac Symposium Paris 1937 (aus Greep in Handbook of Physiology, Endocrinology IV, Part 2, 1974) mit Genehmigung R. O. Greep.

Evans' Methode und zeigte, daß ICSH und LH identisch sind (1937). Die *Evans*-Gruppe beschrieb als erste eine Leydig Zell Atrophie nach Hypophysektomie und der Terminus Interstitial cell-stimulating hormone (ICSH) wurde geprägt (*Evans,* 1937). Die von *van Dyke* und *Coffin* (1941) benutzten Begriffe Thylakentrin für FSH und Metakentrin für ICSH setzten sich nicht durch. „This name (thylakentrin) was introduced ... to refer to pure follicle stimulating hormone whose action appears to be solely to stimulate follicle growth unaccompanied by estrogen secretion unless metakentrin also is administered" (*Greep* et al., 1941).

Ph. E. Smith faßte die Kenntnisse über die Vorderlappenhormone 1935 zusammen: „it is evident that no less than six and possibly eight hormones have been extracted from the anterior pituitary. That this small gland, which in man averages less than 0.5, grams in weight, secretes this number of hormones as separate entities throughout the entire secretory process, taxes the imagination."

Hypothalamus-Hypophysen-Gonadeninteraktion

„Über den Einfluß des Hypophysenvorderlappens auf den Ablauf der Sexualfunktion" lautete 1928 der Titel einer Arbeit von *Hermann Siegmund*, Assistent bei *Emil Knauer* an der Universitäts Frauenklinik Graz. Die Hypothese von *Siegmund* war, daß „der rhythmische Ablauf der Sexualfunktion durch ein antagonistisches Ineinandergreifen von Vorderlappen- und Ovarialhormonen entsteht, indem der auf die Follikelreifung konstant wirkende Reiz des Vorderlappens in bestimmten Zeitabständen von der hemmenden Wirkung der Corpora lutea unterbrochen wird" (*Siegmund*, 1928). *Alfons Mahnert*, ebenfalls in Graz stellte bei Versuchen mit Mäusen fest, daß Hypophysen von Tieren, die mit Transplantaten von Corpora lutea oder mit Östrogenen behandelt worden waren, eine abgeschwächte Wirkung auf die Follikelbildung in den Ovarien infantiler Tiere haben im Vergleich zu Hypophysen unbehandelter Tiere. *Mahnert* folgerte, „daß der vom Hypophysenvorderlappen ausgehende Wachstumsimpuls auf den follikulären Apparat des Ovariums durch das Ovarialhormon zur Zeit seiner größten Produktion (Corpus luteum) gehemmt oder niedergehalten werden kann" (*Mahnert*, 1928). Diese Folgerung kann als erster Hinweis auf einen negativen Feedback der Östrogene auf die Adenohypophyse eingestuft werden.

Den experimentellen Beweis für einen positiven Feedback großer Östrogendosen auf die gonadotrope Funktion des Hypophysenvorderlappen verdanken wir *John C. Burch* und *R. C. Cunningham* von den Departments of Gynecology and of Anatomy, Vanderbilt University in Nashville/Tennessee. Die Transplantation von Hypophysen Östrogen behandelter Tiere führte im Vergleich zu Kontrolltieren zu stärker vergrößerten Ovarien und gesteigerter Vermehrung hämorrhagischer Follikel und Corpora lutea (Burch u. *Cunningham*, 1929).

Die Untersuchungen von *Walter Hohlweg* (*1902 Wien – † 1992 Graz) zur neuroendokrinen Regulation des Hypothalamus-Hypophysenvorderlappen-Gonadensystems haben wesentlich zur Kenntnis der Steuerung endokriner Drüsen beigetragen. Der Chemiker *Hohlweg*, seit 1928 im Hauptlabor

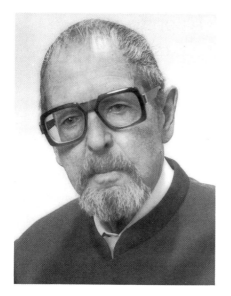

Hohlweg, W. (1902–1992): Chemie-Studium in Wien, Ass. bei Eugen Steinach, 1928 Schering, Berlin, 1931 Leiter der Abt. für Hormonforschung. 1945 Übernahme der Ascheim'schen Abteilung in der Charité, das spätere Institut für experimentelle Endokrinologie. 1961 Graz, Leiter des Hormon-Labors der Frauenklinik. Aufdeckung des Feedback-Mechanismus Hypophyse / Gonaden 1930; Hohlweg-Effekt 1934.

von Schering in Berlin, konnte in Implantationsversuchen zeigen, daß ein Hypophysenvorderlappen mit Kastrationszellen mehr gonadotropes Hormon enthält als Drüsen von nicht kastrierten Tieren. Durch Östrogenzufuhr konnten die histologischen Veränderungen nach der Kastration verhindert, bzw. rückgängig gemacht werden. „Die gonadotrope Funktion des Hypophysenvorderlappen wird durch die hemmende Rückwirkung der Gonadenhormone in physiologischen Grenzen gehalten." Auf dem 2. International Congress for Sex Research am 7. August 1930 in London trug er in seinem Vortrag „Beziehungen zwischen Hypophysenvorderlappen und Keimdrüsen" seine Ergebnisse vor. Die Publikation erfolgte mit *M. Dohrn* (1874–1943), seit 1904 Leiter des physiologischen Labors bei Schering, in den Proceedings des Kongresses 1931 und im Wiener Archiv für Innere Medizin (1930) als Teil einer Festschrift zum 70. Geburtstag von *E. Steinach.* „Man hat sich also vorzustellen, daß normalerweise zwischen Hypophysenvorderlappen und Keimdrüsen quantitative hormonale Beziehungen derart bestehen, daß bestimmte Mengen an Vorderlappenhormon in den Keimdrüsen bestimmte Mengen von Keimdrüsenhormo entstehen lassen und daß durch direkte oder indirekte Rückwirkung der gebildeten Keimdrüsenhormone auf den Vorderlappen, von diesem nur eine begrenzte Menge an Vorderlappenhormon produziert wird."

Aus dem Hauptlaboratorium der Schering-Kahlbaum A.-G., Berlin.

Beziehungen zwischen Hypophysenvorderlappen und Keimdrüsen.*)

Von Dr. **Walter Hohlweg** und Dr. **Max Dohrn**, Berlin.

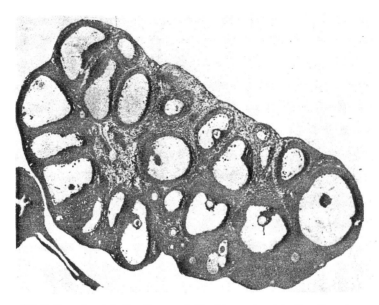

Abb. 5. Ovar einer infantilen Ratte nach Einwirkung einer infantilen Kastraten-
hypophyse. Zahlreiche große Follikel.

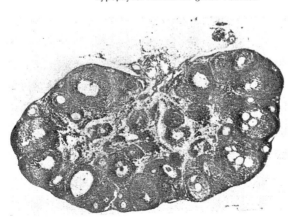

Abb. 6. Ovar einer infantilen Ratte nach Einwirkung der Hypophyse eines mit
Progynon behandelten infantilen Kastraten. Infantiler Zustand.

Hohlweg, W., W. Dohrn: Beziehungen zwischen Hypophysenvorderlappen und Keimdrüsen.
Wiener Arch. Inn. Med. 21 (1930) 337–350. Vortrag London 1930.

Carl R. Moore (*1892 Missouri – † 1955 Chicago) und *Dorothy Price* (*1899 Aurora/Illinois – † 1980 Leiden) vom Department of Zoology der University of Chicago berichteten drei Tage vor *Hohlwegs* Vortrag auf dem gleichen Kongreß entsprechende Befunde („The question of sex hormone antagonism"). Sie hatten gefunden, daß Östrogenextrakte bei Ratten die Gonadotropinsekretion unterdrückten. Alle negativen Wirkungen sind durch Hypophysenvorderlappen-Implantate oder Extrakte zu beheben (*Moore* and *Price,* 1930, 1932). *Ludwig Kraul* an der Universitätsfrauenklinik in Wien untersuchte Hypophysen von Kaninchen, Meerschweinchen und Mäusen, die mit Östrogenen behandelt waren. Wurden diese Hypophysen infantilen Mäusen implantiert, so kommt es zu verstärkten Reaktionen in den Ovarien (*Kraul,* 1931, 1932). Bei erwachsenen Tieren resultieren vermehrt reife Follikel und luteinisierte Follikel.

Die weiteren Untersuchungen waren für Hohlweg der Beweis, daß neben Hypophyse und Gonaden ein Regulationszentrum bestehen muß, das aufgrund des Hormonspiegels im Blut die Funktion der Hypophyse und der Gonaden steuert (Sexualzentrum). Zusammen mit *Karl Junkmann* (* 1897 Leitmeritz – † 1976 Berlin), Leiter des Hauptlabors bei Schering, veröffentlichte er dies in der Klinischen Wochenschrift 1932: „Die innere Sekretion der Keimdrüsen und des Hypophysenvorderlappens wird durch ein nervöses Zentrum beherrscht. Das auf einen bestimmten Sexualhormonspiegel reagierende Sexualzentrum regelt die Tätigkeit der Hypophyse in dem Sinne, daß bei eintretendem Mangel an Sexualhormonen auf nervösem Wege eine verstärkte gonadotrope Vorderlappensekretion zustandekommt, die ihrerseits rein hormonal zur vermehrten Produktion von Keimdrüsenhormon führt. Von der jeweiligen Einstellung des Zentrums wird der Grad der sexuellen Aktivität bestimmt" (*Hohlweg* und *Junkmann,* 1932). Zwei Jahre später hatte *Hohlweg* versucht, durch Vorbehandlung mit Östrogenen eine Atrophie der Ovarien zu erzeugen. Es kam jedoch nicht zur Atrophie, sondern zur Bildung von funktionsfähigen Gelbkörpern. Bei juvenilen Ratten konnte durch Follikelhormoninjektion ebenfalls eine Gelbkörperbildung induziert werden (Hohlweg-Effekt). Die Luteinisierung wurde verhindert, wenn die Tiere zwei Tage nach der Östrogeninjektion hypophysektomiert wurden, während die Corpora lutea sich normal entwickeln, wenn die Hypophysektomie vier Tage nach der Follikelhormoninjektion erfolgt. „Das Resultat dieser Versuche läßt uns erkennen, daß Bildung und Ausschüttung des luteogenen Hormons zwischen dem 2. und 4. Tag nach der Follikelhormoninjektion erfolgen muß. Genau zur selben Zeit, zu der nach Follikelhormonzufuhr der

Oestrus auftritt, reagiert auch der Vorderlappen mit Bildung und Ausschüttung des luteogenen Hormons" (*Hohlweg* u. *Chamorro*, 1937).

Hohlwegs Befunde wurden von *A. Westman* und *Dora Jacobsohn* in der Frauenklinik in Lund bestätigt (1938). *Dora Jacobsohn* war 1934 nach Beendigung des Medizinstudiums in Berlin nach Schweden emigriert. *G. Dörner* (˙ 1929 Hindenburg/Schlesien), der Nachfolger von *Hohlweg* am Institut für experimentelle Endokrinologie in Berlin, und *F. Döcke* zeigten in Rattenversuchen, daß der Hohlweg-Effekt geschlechtsspezifisch weiblich ist (1964).

Axel Westman in Stockholm untersuchte den Einfluß von Hypophysenvorderlappen-Hormonen auf die Funktion des Corpus luteum (1932). „Die Entwicklung und Lebensdauer des normalen Corpus luteum werden weder vom Fehlen, noch vom Vorhandensein einer erhöhten Menge des Hypophysenhormons oder funktionell gleichartiger endokriner Substanzen beeinflußt. Unter diesen Umständen ist kaum anzunehmen, daß eine variierende Funktion der Hypophyse mit abwechselnder Absonderung von Hormon A und B den Sexualzyklus reguliert. Das Vorhandensein beider – sofern sie nun ganz voneinander verschiedene Substanzen sind – ist erforderlich, damit eine Follikelberstung stattfinden kann, wobei der Impuls zu einer normalen Corpus luteum-Bildung gegeben wird. Wenn sich der gelbe Körper aber gut entwickelt hat, funktioniert er selbständig und dient dadurch selbst als Regulator der rhythmischen Variationen in den weiblichen Sexualorganen" (*Westman*, 1932).

Das Gefäßsystem zwischen Hypothalamus und Hypophysenvorderlappen wurde 1930 von *Pietsch* und von *Popa* und *Fielding* beschrieben. Bereits 1742 hatte jedoch *Joseph Lieutaud* in Aix-on-Provence auf die Gefäße, die entlang des Hypophysenstiels laufen und Verbindung zur Hypophyse haben hingewiesen (*Lieutaud*, 1742). Auf diese Beobachtung hat *Sir Solly Zuckerman* in der 7. Addison Memorial Lecture 1953 „The secretion of the brain; relation of hypothalamus to pituitary gland" hingewiesen: „For it so happens that in the course of his studies he stumbled on what is called today the pituitary-portal system" (*Zuckerman*, 1953). *Bernardo Alberto Houssay* (˙1887 Buenos Aires – † 1971 Buenos Aires) erkannte 1935 den „abwärts" gerichteten Blutfluß in den Portalgefäßen. Durch die Untersuchungen von *Wislokki* und *King* (1936) und von *Green* und *Harris* (1947) ergaben sich Hinweise auf eine humorale Transmission durch die Portalgefäße.

1. „The anatomy of the nervous and vascular connexions between the neurohypophysis and adenohypophysis is described.
2. The nervous connexions are scanty in the rabbit, monkey and man.

3. The vascular connexions are prominent in the rat, guinea-pig, rabbit, dog and man. They are described with particular reference to the capillary loops found in the median eminence and infundibular stem, and the hypophysial portal vessels.

4. Nerve fibres from the hypothalamico-hypophyseal tract are intimately associated with the capillary loops.

5. It is suggested that the central nervous system regulates the activity of the adenohypophysis by means of a humoral relay through the hypophysial portal vessels" (*Green* u. *Harris,* 1947).

Geoffrey Wingfield Harris (1913–1971) war Anatom in Cambridge, 1948 Physiologie-Professor, seit 1952 in London, 1962 Anatomieprofessor in Oxford. „A review of *Harris's* work reads like a chapter in the history of endocrinology. The control of multiple activities of the pituitary gland, and the study of the reciprocal interactions of brain and endocrine glands are the topics he has made his own. Step by step *Harris* contributed building stones to our present knowledge, always making sure that his ground was unshakeable before proceeding to the next step. He was one of the founders of the subject of neuroendocrinology" (*Marthe Vogt,* 1972).

1949 erschien die Arbeit von *W. Bargmann* „Über die neurosekretorische Verknüpfung von Hypothalamus und Hypophyse". *Bargmann* (˙1906 Nürnberg – † 1978 Kiel), seit 1942 Anatom in Königsberg, 1946 in Kiel konnte durch experimentelle Durchtrennung des Hypophysenstiels die Transporthypothese sichern. 1952 erbrachten *Geoffrey Wingfield Harris* und *Dora Jacobsohn* (˙1908 Berlin – † 1983 Lund/Schweden) den Beweis dafür, daß die Funktion der Hypophyse nur möglich ist im Kontakt mit dem Hypothalamus. „Our findings agree with this and go further by showing that an animal's own hypophysis, after losing its ability to support ovarian functions other than progestional when the gland is removed from the influence of the tuber cinereum, will regain them when this influence is restored" (*Nikowitch-Winer* and *Everett,* 1958). *F. A. Scharrer, Bertha Scharrer* und *W. Bargmann* entwickelten das Konzept der Bildung neurohypophysärer Hormone in neurosekretorischen Zellen der hypothalamischen Kerngebiete (*Scharrer,* 1954). Die *Scharrers* verließen 1937 Deutschland, obgleich sie nicht von den Machthabern verfolgt wurden, aber sie wollten nicht an der von ihnen vorausgesehenen Entwicklung beteiligt sein. Sie wirkten am Department of Anatomy am Albert Einstein College in New York.

Jacobsohn mußte 1934 Deutschland verlassen, aufgrund des „Arierparagraphen" erfüllte sie nicht die Voraussetzungen für eine medizinische Appro-

THE NEUROVASCULAR LINK BETWEEN THE NEUROHYPOPHYSIS AND ADENOHYPOPHYSIS

By J. D. GREEN and G. W. HARRIS

From the Anatomy School, University of Cambridge

(Received 11 November 1946)

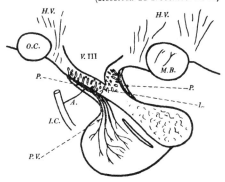

Fig. 2. Diagram of a sagittal section through the hypophysis and hypothalamus to show the general results. The arterial supply to the pars tuberalis is derived from small twigs (*A.*) from the internal carotid artery (*I.C.*). These twigs break up into a rich vascular plexus (*P.*) situated between the pars tuberalis and median eminence. From this plexus are derived vessels which enter the median eminence to form very characteristic sinusoidal loops (*L.*). These loops appear to drain into portal vessels (*P.V.*) which pass into the pars distalis and are distributed to the typical sinuses of this region. The vascular pattern of the median eminence is distinctly different from that of the hypothalamus (*H.V.*) and of the infundibular process. *M.B.* mammillary bodies; *O.C.* optic chiasma; *V. III*, infundibular recess of third ventricle.

SUMMARY

1. The anatomy of the nervous and vascular connexions between the neurohypophysis and adenohypophysis is described.

2. The nervous connexions are scanty in the rabbit, monkey, and man.

3. The vascular connexions are prominent in the rat, guinea-pig, rabbit, dog and man. They are described with particular reference to the capillary loops found in the median eminence and infundibular stem, and the hypophysial portal vessels.

4. Nerve fibres from the hypothalamico-hypophysial tract are intimately associated with the capillary loops.

5. It is suggested that the central nervous system regulates the activity of the adenohypophysis by means of a humoral relay through the hypophysial portal vessels.

Green, J. D., G. W. Harris: The neurovascular link between the neurohypophysis and adenohypophysis. J. Endocrinol. 5 (1947) 136–147 (reproduced by permission of the Journal of Endocrinology Ltd.).

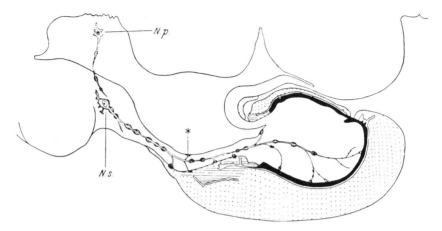

Bargmann, W.: Zwischenhirn und Hypophyse. Arch. Gyn. 183 (1953) 14–34. Abb. 9. (Copyright Springer-Verlag).

bation. Als Jüdin emigrierte sie nach Schweden und arbeitete bei *Axel Westman* in Lund. 1947 begann ihre Zusammenarbeit mit *Harris*.

Der Abteilungsarzt und Prosektor an der Berliner Heil- und Pflegeanstalt Herzberge und Berlin-Wuhlgarten *Franz Josef Kallmann* ('1897 Neumarkt/Schlesien – † 1965 New York) erkannte den Zusammenhang zwischen Anosmie und Hypogonadismus, ein Symptomenkomplex, den schon 1856 *San Juan* beschrieben hatte. *Kallmann* veröffentlichte seine Befunde nach der Emigration in New York (*Kallmann*, 1943, 1944; *San Juan*, 1856). *Schwanzel-Fukuda* et al. entdeckten das Fehlen von LHRH-bildenden Zellen im Hypothalamus. Die Wanderung der LHRH exprimierenden Neurone von der medialen Riechplakode in den medialen Hypothalamus ist beim Kallmann-Syndrom gestört (*Schwanzel-Fukuda* et al., 1989).

Auch *Kallmann* emigrierte 1936 als Jude (considered by the Nazis allthough not by himself) nach New York. Als Psychiater untersuchte er das familiäre Vorkommen einer Anosmie in Verbindung mit einem Hypogonadismus.

An der Aufklärung der Funktion, der Isolierung und Charakterisierung, sowie der Strukturaufklärung der Releasinghormone waren viele Arbeitsgruppen beteiligt. Der Terminus Releasing factor (RF) wurde von *Saffran* 1955 geprägt. *Roger Guillemin* ('1924) benutzte als erster das Adjektiv „hypophysiotrop". *Schally* schlug den Ausdruck hypothalamische Releasinghormone vor und *J. Meites* den Inhibitingfaktor.

1959 *S. M. McCann* „discovered that median eminence extracts from the rat deplete ovarian ascorbic acid in the immature PMS-hCG-primed rat, the most sensitive assay for LH. We continued this work with the arrival of *S. Taleisnik* in the laboratory and published our initial report on LH-releasing factor in 1960. ... Further experiments followed to look for other factors in hypothalamic extracts which release anterior pituitary hormones. *Matsuo Igarashi* (˙ 1925 Tokyo) arrived in the laboratory in 1963 with a mouse uterine weight assay for FSH. After initial work to improve the assay we were able to demonstrate the presence of an FSH-releasing factor in hypothalamic extracts of rat and beef origin" (*McCann*, 1995). In der Pariser Arbeitsgruppe unter der Leitung von *R. Courrier* wurde 1960 mit der Isolierung von LRF durch *Guillemin, Jutisz, Sakiz* und *P. Aschheim* begonnen. 1961 erschien die erste Arbeit über die Charakterisierung von LRF in einem Extrakt von Schaf-Hypothalamus (*Courrier* et al., 1961). *Marian Jutisz* (˙ 1920 in Porohy/Polen) hat die Entwicklung der Forschungen in Paris ausführlich in einem persönlichen Bericht beschrieben (in *Bettendorf*, 1995, S. 274–284). Zwei Arbeitsgruppen konnten 1971 die Aufklärung der Struktur von LH-RH berichten (*Matsuo* et al., 1971 und *Burgos* et al., 1971), es ist ein Decapeptid.

Bestimmungsmethoden von FSH und LH

Eine Vielzahl von biologischen Tests zum qualitativen und quantitativen Nachweis von Gonadotropinen, von FSH und von LH wurden entwickelt. Ein Vergleich der quantitativen Ergebnisse war dadurch erschwert, daß es keine einheitliche Bezugsgröße gab. *Tiereinheiten* beruhen auf dem Nachweis und der Stärke einer spezifischen Reaktion beim Versuchstier. *Li* schlug 1958 vor die Tiereinheiten durch *Slope Einheiten* zu ersetzen: Gewicht des Testorgans minus Gewicht des Kontrollorgans, dividiert durch die verabfolgte Dosis in mg. Die Einführung von Standard- oder Referenz-Präparaten eröffnete die Möglichkeit, zuverlässige und vergleichbare Resultate zu gewinnen. *Borth, Diczfalusy* und *Heinrich* erarbeiteten die Grundlagen zur statistischen Auswertung der biologischen Bestimmungen (1957).

Meilensteine in der Festlegung von Standards waren zwei Konferenzen: 1. Workshop on Gonadotropins, 3.–5. Dezember 1959 in Gatlinburg, Tennessee und 2. The Problem of the International Reference Preparation, eine Woche vor dem 1. Internationalen Endokrinologen Kongreß am 24. Juli 1960 in Kopenhagen (Human Pituitary Gonadotropins, a workshop conference. ed. *A. Albert, Ch. C. Thomas,* Springfield/Illinois, 1961). Bei der Conference on the Standardization of Sex-Hormones 1938 in Genf unter dem Vorsitz von *Sir Henry Dale* war Übereinstimmung erzielt worden für Standards für hCG, PMS und Prolaktin, aber nicht für die Gonadotropine (*Parkes,* 1965).

Der Aschheim-Zondek Test zum Schwangerschaftsnachweis, d.h. zur hCG-Messung wurde bereits erwähnt. *Maurice H. Friedman* vom Department of Physiology, University of Pennsylvania zeigte, daß die Injektion von Schwangerenurin zur Bildung von Corpora haemorrhagica im Kaninchen-Ovar führt und dieser Effekt zum Nachweis einer Gravidität benutzt werden kann (1929). „Non pregnant rabbit does were injected intraperitoneally with 12 cc. of fresh catheter urine from pregnant women, twice daily for four days. On the sixth day, the injected animals were killed and their ovaries removed for examination. In every ovary large, fresh corpora lutea were seen."

THE QUANTITATIVE ASSAY OF "FOLLICLE STIMULATING" SUBSTANCES[1]

LOUIS LEVIN[2] AND H. H. TYNDALE

From the Department of Anatomy, College of Physicians and Surgeons, Columbia University

NEW YORK CITY

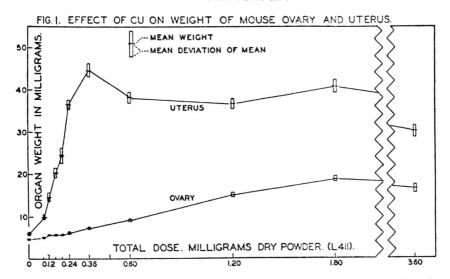

FIG. I. EFFECT OF CU ON WEIGHT OF MOUSE OVARY AND UTERUS.

Levin, L., H. H. Tyndale: The quantitative assay of „Follicle stimulating" substances. (© Endocrine Society) Endocrinology 21 (1937) 619–628.

Louis Levin und *H. H. Tyndale* am Department of Anatomy der Columbia University in New York beschrieben 1937 den Maus-Uterus-Test. Mit diesem Test wird die FSH und LH Aktivität erfaßt (Gesamtgonadotropin). „Assay of FSH-potency on the basis of the weight response of the mouse ovary involves a possible error of at least 100 per cent. The weight of the mouse uterus is relatively and absolutely a very sensitive indicator of FSH-potency and affords a simple, accurate criterion for quantitative assay."

R. O. Greep verdanken wir den Prostatalappen-Test: „in 1941 we found that the LH-induced increase in weight of the anterior prostate of hypophysectomized immature male rats could be used as a quantitative bioassay of LH. The chief advantages in using the anterior prostate in the assay of metakentrin are:

1. The assay can be read objectively.
2. The assay can be placed on a quantitative basis.

12092

Use of Anterior Lobe of Prostate Gland in the Assay of Metakentrin.

R. O. Greep, H. B. van Dyke and Bacon F. Chow.

From the Division of Pharmacology, the Squibb Institute for Medical Research, New Brunswick, N.J.

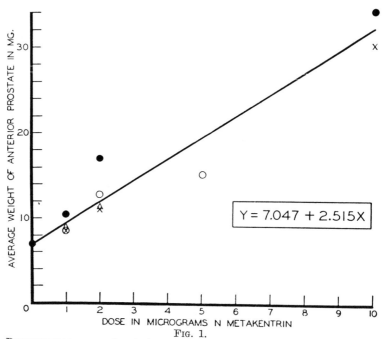

Fig. 1.

Dose-response curve of anterior prostate of hypophysectomized immature rats receiving total doses of 1-10 μg of N of pure metakentrin of which one-fourth was administered daily for 4 days. See also text.

Greep, R. O., H. B. van Dyke, B. F. Chow: Use of anterior lobe of prostate gland in the assay of metakentrin. Proc. Soc. Exp. Biol. Med. 46 (1941) 644–649 (with permission of R. O. Greep).

3. No histological preparations or evaluations are required.

4. The presence of thylakentrin does not influence the assay" (*Greep, Dyke, Chow, 1941, Greep* et al., 1942, *Greep,* 1995).

Evans benutzte „a technique employing the repair of interstitial cells of the hypophysectomized immature female ovary as an assay for ICSH" (*Evans* et al., 1939). *Bradbury* machte die Beobachtung, daß Gonadotropine bereits in kleinen Dosen eine Hyperämie der Ovarien hervorrufen und entwickelte daraus einen Test zur Mengenbestimmung (1944). *Parlow* und *Reichert* (1963) überprüften den von *S. Ells* 1961 publizierten Ovar-Hyperämie-Test für LH. Die Hyperämie wurde mit jodmarkiertem Serum Albumin gemessen. Für Schaf-LH war die Methode empfindlicher als der Prostatalappentest und auch als der OAAD-Test.

Das gebräuchlichste Verfahren zur Messung von FSH war lange Zeit der *Steelman* und *Pohley* Assay. Dieser Augmentationstest beruht auf der Beobachtung, daß hCG die Wirkung von FSH am Ovar verstärkt. Als Testtiere werden entweder Ratten (*Steelman/Pohley*, 1953) oder Mäuse (*Brown*, 1955) benutzt.

Nachdem *Sayers* et al. 1948 einen Ascorbinsäureabfall in den Nebennieren nach Einwirkung von kortikotropem Hormon beschrieben hatte und diese Reaktion als Test für die ACTH-Wirkung eingesetzt wurde, untersuchte *Heinrich Karg* (* 1928 München) am Institut für Physiologie und Ernährung der Tiere in München Ascorbinsäurewerte im Ovar nach gonadotroper Stimulation. *Hökfelt* hatte 1949 einen Vitamin-C-Abfall nach Gonadotropinen im Ovar gefunden. In der Arbeit „Ascorbinsäuredynamik im Ovar als Gonadotropinnachweis", beschrieb *Karg* 1957 das Prinzip des später so benannten Ovarian-Ascorbic-Acid-Depletion Test (OAAD). Er konnte zeigen, daß LH und hCG bei Ratten einen temporären, Dosis-abhängigen Ascorbinsäureabfall in den Ovarien bewirkt. Ein Jahr später publizierte *A. Parlow* seinen OAAD-Test (*Parlow*, 1958).

Eine spezifische und sehr empfindliche Methode zur FSH-Bestimmung wurde von *Igarashi* und *McCann* auf dem Endocrine Society meeting in Atlantic City vorgetragen (1963). Sie basiert auf dem Synergismus von FSH und geringen Mengen von hCG. An drei Tagen wird das zu testende Material zusammen mit 0,25 IU oder 0,1 IU hCG immaturen weiblichen Mäusen injiziert. An Tag 4 dient das Uterusgewicht als Maß der FSH-Aktivität (*Igarashi* and *McCann*, 1964).

Ein sensitiver Bioassay für Serum-LH und hCG basierend auf der Testosteronbildung isolierter Ratten-Leydigzellen auf eine Gonadotropinstimulation wurde im NIH entwickelt (*Dufau* et al., 1976).

Von Damme et al. (1979) beschrieben einen FSH in vitro bioassay mit Sertolizellen. Der Methode liegt das von *Dorrington* (1976) beschriebene Prinzip der Östradiolproduktion aus 19-hydroxyandrostendion abhängig von der FSH-Konzentration zugrunde.

1934 hat *Collip* die Bildung von Antihormonen im Sinne von Antikörpern nach Injektion artfremder Proteohormone berichtet. Nach der Beobachtung, daß hCG zur Bildung von Antikörpern führt und damit durch eine

ASSAY OF THE FOLLICLE STIMULATING HORMONE BASED ON THE AUGMENTATION WITH HUMAN CHORIONIC GONADOTROPIN

SANFORD L. STEELMAN AND FLORENCE M. POHLEY

From the Fundamental Research Department, The Armour Laboratories and the Research Division, Armour and Company, Chicago, Illinois

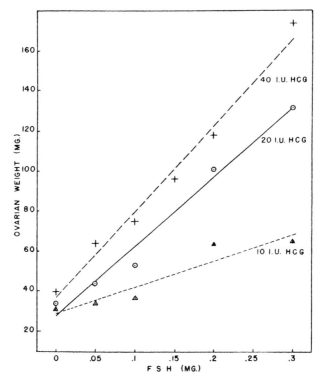

FIG. 1. Regression lines for assays of FSH augmented by 10, 20, and 40 I.U. of HCG.

Steelman, S. L., F. M. Pohley: Assay of the follicle stimulating hormone based on the augmentation with human chorionic gonadotropin. (© Endocrine Society) Endocrinology 153 (1953) 604–616

reifen Sprague-Dawley-Ratten von 120—150 g Gewicht, deren Cyclus in einer Vorperiode kontrolliert worden war, wurde CG subcutan verabreicht. Die Ascorbinsäurebestimmungen wurden nach dem von uns modifizierten[6] colorimetrischen Verfahren vorgenommen, um in einem Arbeitsgang gleichzeitig neben der Ovarascorbinsäure auch den Ascorbinsäure- und Adrenalingehalt der Nebennieren miterfassen zu können. Versuche hinsichtlich des zeitlichen Ablaufes der CG-Wirkung ergaben maximale Erniedrigung der Ascorbinsäuregehalte der Ovarien nach etwa 8 Std (Tabelle 1). Auf diese Einwirkungsdauer wurde der in Tabelle 2 wiedergegebene Versuch mit unterschiedlichen CG-Dosierungen (bezogen jeweils auf 100 g Körpergewicht) eingestellt. Es konnten gut gesicherte Wirkungsunterschiede zwischen den einzelnen Gruppen (Gruppengröße nur 6—10 Ratten!) gefunden werden. Als Bezugswert für die Angabe des prozentualen Ascorbinsäureabfalls diente eine diöstrische Kontrollgruppe. Der Wert einer östrischen Kontrollgruppe entsprach annähernd dem 8 Std-Wert bei 5 E CG, was einen

Tabelle 1. *Wirkung von 100 E Choriongonadotropin auf Ovarascorbinsäure in Abhängigkeit von der Zeit*

Stunden nach CG	Ascorbinsäuregehalt Ovar mg-%	Ascorbinsäuregehalt Ovar in % gegen Ausgangswert
0	91,3 ± 3,4	100
1	72,7 ± 2,0	80
2	56,4 ± 2,1	62
4	45,2 ± 2,4	49
8	38,3 ± 1,6	42
12	50,0 ± 3,8	55
24	66,2 ± 3,8	72

Tabelle 2. *Wirkung von Choriongonadotropin auf Ovarascorbinsäure nach 8 Std in Abhängigkeit von der Dosis*

CG-Dosis E	Ascorbinsäuregehalt Ovar mg-%	Ascorbinsäuregehalt Ovar in % gegen Ausgangswert
0 (diöstrisch)	91,3 ± 3,4	100
0 (östrisch)	69,0 ± 3,1	76
5	67,4 ± 2,2	74
10	54,6 ± 1,1	60
20	48,0 ± 1,3	53
100	38,3 ± 1,6	42

Rückschluß auf die endogene physiologische Dosis zuläßt. Die Wirkungsspezifität entnehmen wir daraus, daß durch ACTH ebensowenig die Ovarascorbinsäure beeinflußt wurde, wie andererseits der Vitamin C-Gehalt der Nebennieren durch CG sich nicht signifikant veränderte. Demnach könnte die Prüfung auf gonadotrope Wirksamkeit an cycluskontrollierten Ratten auch ohne Hypophysektomie erfolgen. Es sei noch auf den prinzipiellen zeitlichen Wirkungsunterschied des CG gegenüber dem ACTH am Erfolgsorgan hingewiesen (Minimum der Nebennierenascorbinsäure im Sayers-Test nach einer Stunde). Die feststellbare maximale Erniedrigung der Drüsenascorbinsäure auf etwa 42% des Normalwertes zeigt jedoch eine auffallende Übereinstimmung (s. [7]).

Die Arbeit konnte dank der Unterstützung der Deutschen Forschungsgemeinschaft durchgeführt werden.

ASCORBINSÄUREDYNAMIK IM OVAR ALS GONADOTROPINNACHWEIS

Von

Heinrich Karg

(Eingegangen am 2. Mai 1957)

Aus dem Institut für Physiologie und Ernährung der Tiere der Universität München (Vorstand: Prof. Dr. Dr. Johannes Brüggemann)

Der Befund des Ascorbinsäureabfalls in den Nebennieren nach Einwirkung von corticotropem Hormon[1] hat als Standardtest für ACTH, als Kriterium in zahlreichen Stressversuchen bis hin zu der Frage der Ascorbinsäurebeteiligung bei der Corticosteroidbiosynthese[2] starke Beachtung gefunden. Entsprechende Ascorbinsäureuntersuchungen im Ovar nach gonadotroper Stimulierung stehen noch aus; lediglich Hökfelt[3] weist auf Vitamin C-Abfall in den interstitiellen Zellen des Kaninchenovars nach Gonadotropin hin, und Coste[4] führte Befunde von Cyclusschwankungen der Ovarascorbinsäure auf die glandotrope Hormonwirkung zurück. Eigene Untersuchungen erstreckten sich zunächst auf die Zeit-Dosis-Beziehungen der Wirkung von Choriongonadotropin (CG)[5] auf den Ascorbinsäuregehalt von Rattenovarien. Geschlechts-

Literatur. [1] Sayers, M. A., G. Sayers and L. A. Woodbury: Endocrinology **42**, 379 (1948). — [2] Kersten, H., W. Kersten u. H. J. Staudinger: Biochem. Z. **328**, 24 (1956). — [3] Claesson, L., N. Hillarp, B. Högberg u. B. Hökfelt: Acta endocrinol. (Copenh.) **2**, 249 (1949). — [4] Coste, F., F. Delbarre et F. Lacronique: C. r. Soc. Biol. Paris **147**, 611 (1953). — [5] *Primogonyl*, von der Fa. Schering, Berlin, freundlicherweise zur Verfügung gestellt. — [6] Brüggemann, J., H. Karg u. O. Käppeler: Vitamine u. Hormone **7**, 200 (1956). — [7] Karg, H.: Z. physiol. Chem. **304**, 148 (1956).

A New Sensitive Bio-assay for Follicle-Stimulating Hormone (FSH)

M. IGARASHI[1] AND S. M. McCANN

Department of Physiology, School of Medicine, University of Pennsylvania, Philadelphia, Pennsylvania

ABSTRACT. A specific and very sensitive assay method for FSH using intact immature female mice was devised. This method is based on the synergism between FSH and a small amount of human chorionic gonadotrophin (HCG). The test material mixed together with 0.25 IU or 0.1 IU HCG is injected subcutaneously daily for 3 days into intact immature female mice. On the fourth day, necropsy is performed and uterine weight is measured after evacuation of any fluid. Using NIH-FSH and IRP-HMG, linear log-dose response curves were obtained. By contrast, the ovine NIH-LH standard evoked no significant

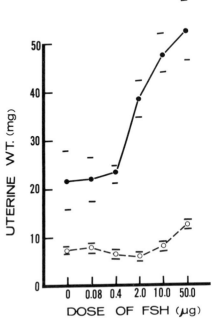

FIG. 1. Effect of varying doses of FSH (logarithmic scale) on mouse uterine weight. — — ○ represents the mean uterine weight in mice which received only FSH, whereas ——— ● represents the uterine weight in mice treated with 0.25 IU of HCG, and varying doses of FSH. The dashes above and below each point represent the standard error of the mean.

SEVERAL methods for the assay of follicle-stimulating hormone (FSH) have been devised and used; however, most of them are complicated and relatively insensitive. Steelman-Pohley's (1) and P. S. Brown's (2) methods are being applied widely since they are easy to carry out and are specific for FSH, but these two methods suffer from a lack of sensitivity. Among the various bio-assay methods for gonadotrophins, the mouse uterine weight method has been recognized as the most sensitive assay by several workers (3–7), but it is not only nonspecific for FSH, but also still too insensitive to assay small amounts of gonadotrophin. In order to obtain a

Received August 28, 1963.
This work was supported by NIH Grant No. A-1236, C-6, and by a grant from the Population Council for Dr. Igarashi's laboratory expenses.

[1] Fellow of the Population Council, on leave from the Department of Obstetrics and Gynecology, Gunma University Medical School, Maebashi, Japan.

[2] NIH-FSH-S-1 ovine standard.
[3] NIH-LH-S-3 ovine standard.
[4] Kindly provided by National Institute for Medical Research, London.
[5] Kindly provided by Dr. John B. Jewell of Ayerst Laboratories.

Igarashi, M., S. M. McCann: A new sensitive bio-assay for follicle-stimulating hormone (FSH).
(© Endocrine Society) Endocrinology 74 (1964) 440–445.

In Vitro Bioassay of LH in Human Serum: The Rat Interstitial Cell Testosterone (RICT) Assay

M. L. DUFAU, R. POCK, A. NEUBAUER, AND K. J. CATT

Section on Hormonal Regulation, Reproduction Research Branch, National Institute of Child Health and Human Development, National Institutes of Health, Bethesda, Maryland 20014

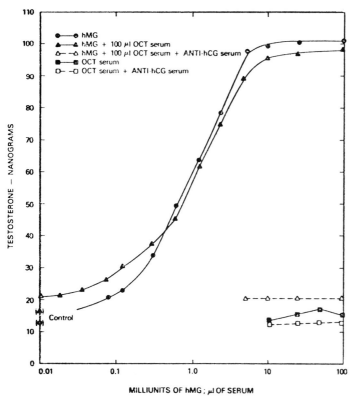

FIG. 1. Testosterone response curves obtained by the incubation of rat interstitial cells with increasing concentrations of standard gonadotropin (hMG) in the presence or absence of gonadotropin-free serum, and in the presence of anti-hCG serum. Although the effect of added serum was relatively small in this example, the addition of gonadotropin-free serum or 5% BSA was necessary during routine use of the assay to ensure the homogeneity of standard curves and dose-response curves of the serum samples.

Dufau, M. L., R. Pock, A. Neubauer, K. J. Catt: In vitro bioassay of LH in human serum: the rat interstitial cell testosterone (RICT) assay. J. Clin. Endocrinol. Metabol. 42 (1976) 958–969.

Antigen-Antikörper Reaktion nachgewiesen kann, wurden zur Bestimmung der hormonellen Aktivität die immunologischen Tests entwickelt. *Brody* u. *Carlström* (1960, 1961) wählten für die quantitative Bestimmung von hCG den Komplement-Fixations-Test. *Wide* fand eine Hemmung der Hämagglutination zwischen anti-hCG-sera und hCG-coated Blutzellen durch humanes LH. Er entwickelte einen Test zur immunologischen Bestimmung von LH aus Hypophysen und aus Urin (*Wide* et al., 1961) und 1960 zusammen mit *Gemzell* den ersten immunologischen hCG-Test (Pregnosticon) „The method ist based upon the inhibition of haemagglutination reaction of stable hCG coated blood cells (hCG-cells) in the presence of hCG-antiserum"; 1961 den ersten Immuno-Assay für hLH; 1966–1968 den kompetitiven solid-phase immunoassay und die nonkompetitive „sandwich" Technik. Die immunologische Methode erlaubte auch die Bestimmung von Gonadotropin in Nichtschwangeren Urin (*Breckwoldt*, 1966). Durch Verdünnungsreihen war es möglich, die Gonadotropinausscheidung semiquantitativ zu ermitteln. *Niswender* entwickelte einen Radioimmunoassay für LH (*Niswender* et al., 1968). Der in einem Kaninchen produzierte Antikörper gegen bovines LH zeigte eine Kreuzreaktion mit anderen Spezies. Mit dem von *Parlow* hergestellten Antikörper für Ratten-LH fand sich eine gute Übereinstimmung zwischsen Bioassay (OAAD) und Immunoassay (*Bogdanove* et al., 1971).

Mit dem RIA war es möglich geworden Bestimmungen in kleinsten Proben mit großer Genauigkeit durchzuführen. Ein Vergleich der Ergebnisse mit denen von biologischen Methoden ergaben jedoch Diskrepanzen. *Von Damme* entwickelte einen LH in vitro bioassay auf der Basis einer Testosteronsekretion von Maus-Leydig Zellen (*Von Damme* et al., 1979). Auf die Probleme, die bei Messungen von Serumproben auftreten, haben *Lichtenberg* (1980) und *Lichtenberg* u. *Pahnke* (1976) hingewiesen. Die spezifischen LH-Rezeptorbindung an Ratten-Leydigzellmembranen wurde das Prinzip des von *Leidenberger* und *Reichert* (1972) und *von Catt* et al. (1972) beschriebenen Rezeptorassay. *Bhalla* und *Reichert* (1974) benutzten die FSH-Rezeptorbindung an Ratten-Tubulifraktionen zum in vitro FSH Nachweis.

Gonadotropine in Urin und in Plasma

C. F. Fluhmann (1929) an der Stanford University wies als erster gonadotrope Aktivität im Blut nach. 3–5 ml Serum ovariektomierter Frauen führten bei infantilen Mäusen zu einer Follikelreifung und Bildung von Corpora lutea. Die Einteilung der Ovarreaktionen erfolgte nach den von *Zondek* und *Aschheim* angegebenen Kategorien. Bei 12 von 19 Patienten nach Ovarektomie war die Reaktion positiv, ebenso bei fünf nach Radiumkastration. 6 von 17 Patienten mit einer funktionellen Amenorrhö und drei von fünf mit irregulären Blutungen „showed anterior pituitary hormone in the blood."

Janet W. McArthur (1958) bestimmte LH- und FSH-Aktivität in menopausalem Plasma und in Cohns Fraktionen. Beide Aktivitäten waren in allen Fraktionen nachweisbar, FSH konzentriert in Fraktion V und VI (Albumin und Überstand) und LH in Fraktion II und III (δ- und β-Globulin). Dies galt als Hinweis dafür, daß eine partielle Trennung der beiden Aktivitäten erfolgt war.

Für die Extraktion von gonadotroper Aktivität aus dem Urin wurden vor allem die von *Albert* (1956) und die von *Loraine* und *Brown* (1956) angegebene Kaolin-Aceton-Methode benutzt. Beide Methoden wurden von *Heinrichs* und *Eulenfeld* (1960) miteinander verglichen. „Mit der Methode *Albert* wird ein etwa dreifach stärker konzentrierter, untoxischer Extrakt mit einem höheren Gehalt von gonadotroper Aktivität pro Liter bei geringem Zeitaufwand gewonnen. Die technisch vereinfachte Kaolin-Aceton-Methode nach *Albert* wird allen Anforderungen gerecht, die an eine optimale Extraktionsmethode zu stellen sind. Sie kann daher für die Extraktion von HPG aus Urin bei klinischen Routineuntersuchungen und auch bei wissenschaftlichen Fragestellungen verwendet werden." Zur Bestimmung des HPG wurde die Uterus-Gewichtsmethode benutzt. Auf die jahreszeitlichen Schwankungen in der Reaktion der Testtiere wurde hingewiesen und auf die Notwendigkeit einer gleichzeitigen Testung eines Standardpräparates bei jeder biologischen Bestimmung. Beim Vergleich der Alkoholfällungsmethode und der Kaolin-Aceton-Methode erwies sich die erste in bezug auf Ausbeute und wegen der Toxizität der Extrakte unterlegen bzw. ungeeignet (*Keller*, 1963). Zur Extraktion der Gonadotropine aus dem Harn wurde auch die Ultrafiltration eingesetzt (*Gorbman*, 1945, *Schneider* u. *Frahm*, 1961).

M. Apostolakis wies auf die Bedeutung eines Referenz-Standards hin (1960). ICSH wurde mit Hilfe des Prostatalappentests und FSH mit dem HCG-Augmentationstest im Plasma von Menopause-Frauen und Männern nachgewiesen. 1965 beschrieben *Keller* und *Rosemberg* eine Extraktionsmethode, die auch zum quantitativen Nachweis im Plasma von Frauen geeignet erschien. Es wurde FSH und LH im Plasma junger Männer und Frauen in der Menopause bestimmt (*Keller*, 1966).

Die erste Studie über die renale Clearance der hypophysären Gonadotropine wurde 1960 durch *Apostolakis* und *Loraine* vorgelegt. Der mittlere Clearancewert, gemessen aufgrund der gonadotropen Gesamtaktivität, betrug bei postmenopausalen Frauen 0,18 ml / min, von hCG im Vergleich 0,95 ml / min. Nach Verabreichung von hypophysärem Gonadotropin fand sich 10 bis 15 % der verabreichten Menge im Urin. „An appreciable amount beeing present up to three days following the final injection" (*Apostolakis* et al., 1961).

Über die Gonadotropinausscheidung während des ovariellen Zyklus und bei pathologischen Zuständen gab es lange Zeit differierende Befunde. *P. S. Brown* in Birmingham bestimmte 1956 bei amenorrhoischen Frauen die Gonadotropine im Urin mit Hilfe des Maus Uterus Tests (Gesamt-Gonadotropine) und mit der Ovargewichtszunahme bei hCG-behandelten Mäusen

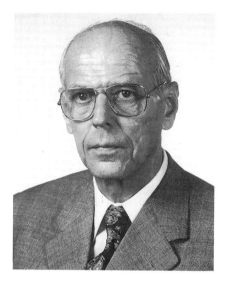

Buchholz, R. (1914 – 1994): Gynäkologe in Düssedorf und Marburg. 1955 LH Maximum zur Zyklusmitte; Wirkung der Steroide auf die Hypophysenfunktion; positiver Feedback von Progesteron.

Zeitschrift für die gesamte experimentelle Medizin, Bd. 128, S. 219—242 (1957)

Aus der Frauenklinik der Medizinischen Akademie Düsseldorf
(Direktor: Prof. Dr. med. H. R. Schmidt-Elmendorff)

Untersuchungen über die Ausscheidungsverhältnisse der gonadotropen Hypophysenhormone FSH und ICSH im mensuellen Cyclus

Von

Rudolf Buchholz

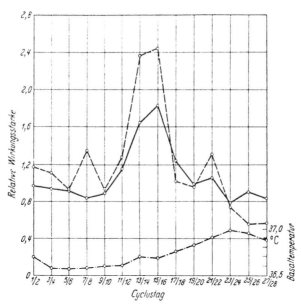

Abb. 6. Graphische Darstellung der relativen Wirkungsstärke der Aktivität der Gesamt-
gonadotropine (o······o) und des ICSH (o————o) an den einzelnen Cyclustagen

Buchholz, R.: Untersuchungen über die Ausscheidungsverhältnisse der gonadotropne Hypophysenhormone FSH und ICSH im menstruellen Zyklus. Z. ges. exp. Med. 128 (1957) 219–242
(mit Genehmigung).

THE URINARY EXCRETION OF OESTROGENS, PREGNANEDIOL AND GONADOTROPHINS DURING THE MENSTRUAL CYCLE

By J. B. BROWN, A. KLOPPER* AND J. A. LORAINE

From the Clinical Endocrinology Research Unit (Medical Research Council), University of Edinburgh

(*Received* 13 *May* 1958)

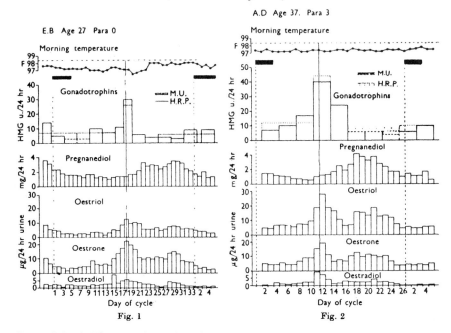

Fig. 1   Fig. 2

Brown, J. B., A. Klopper, J. A. Loraine: The urinary excretion of oestrogens, pregnanediol and gonadotrophins during the menstrual cycle. J. Endocrinology 17 (1958) 401–410 (reproduced with permission of the Journal of Endocrinology Ltd. and J. B. Brown).

(FSH). „The results provide evidence that FSH and ICSH exist as separate entities in human urine."

Rudolf Buchholz (1914 Glogau / Oder – 1994 Marburg) in der Frauenklinik der Medizinischen Akademie in Düsseldorf bestimmte in einem Urinkollektiv von 17 gesunden, geschlechtsreifen Frauen mit regelmäßigem Zyklus die Gesamtgonadotropine mit dem Maus Uterus Test und ICSH mit dem ventralen Prostatatest bei hypophysektomierten Ratten. Beide Kurven zeigten während des ganzen Zyklus einen gleichsinnigen Verlauf mit einem deutlich ausgeprägten Ausscheidungsgipfel um die Zyklusmitte. „Ein Zusammenhang zwischen dem Ausscheidungsgipfel der gonadotropen Hormone und der Ovulation scheint damit gegeben zu sein" (*Buchholz,* 1957).

Borth, Lunenfeld und *de Watteville* untersuchten 6 Zyklen von 5 gesunden Frauen (1957) „Both the gonadotrophin and the estrone peaks coincided with, or preceded, but never occured after, the appearance of pregnanediol."

Brown, Klopper und *Loraine* (1958) benutzten den Maus Uterus Test und den ventralen Prostata-Test hypophysektomierter Ratten. „The pattern of hormone excretion was relatively constant from one individual to another, but the actual amounts excreted varied considerably in different individuals. In none of the subjects studied did the mid-cycle peak in gonadotrophin precede the oestrogen peak. The increase in urinary pregnanediol during the luteal phase occured at the same time as or just before the rise in basal temperature and 1−4 days after the oestrogen peak. When gonadotrophin assays were conducted by the mouse uterus test and that depending on the prostate of the hypophysectomized rat, the results agreed very closely at all stages of the cycle."

Ähnliche Befunde wurden von *J. W. McArthur* und Mitarbeitern in der Harvard Medical School in Boston erhoben (1958). „The findings were as follows: a- In 12 pre-pubertal children, urinary ICSH activity was barely detectable in 3 instances. b- In 5 adult females, ICSH activity was detectable in mid-cycle and in 3 of the 5 subjects it was detectable during the follicular and luteal phase as well. There was no appreciable difference between the excretion rate of ICSH during in the follicular and luteal phases. However, during mid-cycle a twofold to fourfold increase in ICSH activity occured. c- In 17 adult males, ICSH activity was detectable in 16 instances. Although the results were variable, it appeared that males excreted appreciable more ICSH than adult females, except when the latter were in the mid-cycle peak phase of the menstrual cycle. d- In 10 postmenopausal women, the rate of excretion of ICSH was higher than that observed in any other group of either sex." Bei PCO-Patienten fanden sich erhöhte LH-Konzentrationen (1959).

Timing of Ovulation by LH Assay

Melvin L. Taymor, M.D.

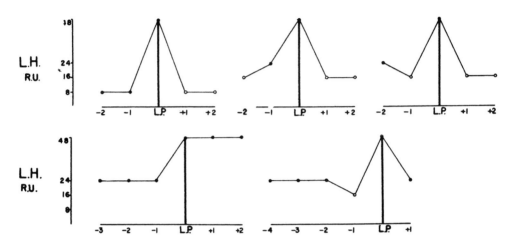

L.P.- LOW POINT ON TEMPERATURE CHART

Fig. 1. Urinary LH excretion at midcycle in 5 cases in which peak excretion coincided with the low point of the temperature chart.

Taymor, M. L.: Timing of ovulatrion by LH assay. Fertil. Steril. 10 (1959) 212–226. Reproduced with permission of the publisher, the American Society for Reproductive Medicine (formerly The American Fertility Society).

Melvin L. Taymor im Peter Bent Brigham Hospital in Boston beschrieb einen „midcycle peak of LH excretion" bei zehn Frauen, „with the hope, that this may produce the physiologic foundation for a practical clinical test for the prediction of ovulation" (*Taymor,* 1959). *Würteler* und *Schmidt* (1959) führten die um den Ovulationstermin gefundenen erhöhten Gonadotropinwerte auf das Hinzukommen von ICSH zu FSH zurück. In gleicher Weise kommentierte auch *Hammerstein* den intermenstruellen Gonadotropin-Anstieg als Folge einer vermehrten LH-Bildung (*Hammerstein,* 1962). In beiden Studien wurde die Klinefelter-Methode benutzt.

Taymor untersuchte Extrakte von Urinpools aus der Follikelphase und mitzyklisch mit dem Ziel, „to demonstrate two separate urinary moieties. It was concluded that there was a qualitative difference in urinary gonadotropin excretion in the two phases of the menstrual cycle studied" (*Taymor,* 1961).

In der gleichen Zeit erschienen die wenig beachteten Arbeiten von *F. Hoffmann* über die hormonale Regulation der Follikelreifung im Zyklus der Frau (1961) und über die Wirkung des Progesterons auf das Follikelwachstum und seine Bedeutung für die hormonale Steuerung des Ovarialzyklus (1962). *Hoffmann* stellte fest, daß eine intraovarielle Injektion von Östradiol oder von Progesteron zu einer Hemmung der Follikelreifung und Verschiebung der Ovulation führt und folgerte daraus, daß ein auf das Ovar begrenzter und von hypophysären Regulationsvorgängen unabhängiger Wirkungseffekt existiert.

Fukushima und Mitarbeiter (1964) bestimmten FSH mit dem Augmentationstest nach *Steelman* und *Pohley* und LH mit dem OAAD-Test nach *Parlow* bei fünf Frauen über elf Zyklen. „There was a consistent pattern of FSH and LH excretion in all cycles studied. The excretion of FSH was highest during the menses and reached a low point at mid-cycle. The greatest effect of estrogen on the vaginal smear occured around mid-cycle and all subjects showed a rise in basal body temperature after the peak excretion of LH activity. The ratio of urinary FSH to LH activity varied significantly during the cycle."

Die zeitliche Korrelation zwischen Gonadotropin- und Östrogenmaxima wurden von *R. Kaiser* et al. in der Frauenklinik in München bestimmt (1964). Die größte Gonadotropinausscheidung gemessen im Mausuterus Test bei fünf Frauen fand sich in jedem Einzelzyklus im 48 Stunden-Sammelharn, der dem Basaltemperaturanstieg vorausging. Die Östrogenmaxima lagen am letzten oder vorletzten Tag des Temperaturtiefs.

Kenneth L. Becker und *A. Albert* an der Mayo Clinic untersuchten die FSH- und LH-Ausscheidung bei endokrinen Erkrankungen mit erhöhten Gonadotropinwerten. „In Turner's syndrome the FSH and LH increased proportionally; hence, the FSH/LH ratio was similar to that of postmenopausal women. A slightly disproportionate increase in FSH and LH excretions in Klinefelter's syndrome raised the FSH/LH ratio to 2.8. The most disproportionate increase was found in castrated men: the excretion of FSH was increased 3-fold but the LH excretion was slightly reduced; hence, the FSH/LH ratio was about 7." FSH wurde im Augmentationstest gegen den Standard NIH-FSH-S1 und LH im ventralen Prostatalappentest gegen NIH-LH gemessen (*Becker* und *Albert,* 1965).

In all diesen Arbeiten wird die Bedeutung der Assay-Methode und die Verwendung der verschiedenen Standards diskutiert. *Eugenia Rosemberg* und

Urinary FSH and LH Excretion During the Normal Menstrual Cycle

MINEKO FUKUSHIMA, M.D.,[1] VERNON C. STEVENS, PH.D.,
CLARENCE L. GANTT, M.D.,[2] AND NICHOLS VORYS, M.D.

Department of Obstetrics and Gynecology and The Division of Endocrinology and Metabolism of The Department of Medicine, The Ohio State University Health Center, Columbus, Ohio

ABSTRACT. The urinary excretion of FSH and LH, as assayed by the ovarian weight augmentation and ovarian ascorbic acid depletion methods and compared with NIH-FSH and LH ovine pituitary standards, was measured throughout 11 menstrual cycles in 5 normal female subjects. Daily vaginal smears were taken as an index of estrogen activity, and basal body temperatures were taken as an index of progesterone effect. There was a consistent pattern of FSH and LH excretion in all cycles studied. The excretion of FSH was highest during the menses and reached a low point at mid-cycle. Significant urinary LH activity was present only at mid-cycle.

The greatest effect of estrogen on the vaginal smear occurred around mid-cycle and all subjects showed a rise in basal body temperature after the peak excretion of LH activity. The ratio of urinary FSH to LH activity varied significantly during the cycle. (*J Clin Endocr* **24**: 205, 1964)

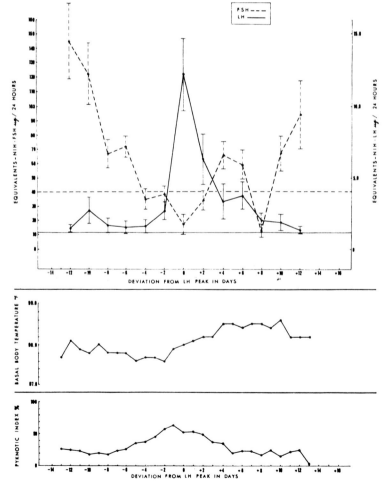

FIG. 7. Mean urinary excretion of FSH (10 cycles) and LH (8 cycles) activity; mean basal body temperatures and mean pyknotic indices arranged according to the deviations from the time of maximal LH excretion in each cycle. The vertical lines about each point represent the standard error. The dashed and solid horizontal lines represent the minimum values for FSH and LH, respectively, which could be distinguished from zero.

Fukushima, M., V. C. Stevens, C. L. Gantt, N. Vorys: Urinary FSH and LH excretion during the normal menstrual cycle. (© the Endocrine Society). J. Clin. Endocrinol. 24 (1964) 205–213.

Paul J. Keller stellten 1965 fest, „the present data confirm those of other workers in suggesting that there is an increase in LH excretion occuring at about midcycle. Whether FSH excretion simply fluctuates throughout the cycle and / or is higher at the beginning and lower at mid-cycle is at present uncertain" (*Rosemberg* and *Keller,* 1965). *Rocca* und *Albert* schlossen aus FSH-Messungen bei 23 Frauen: „Thus, although considerable variation in individual titers was found among different subjects, the FSH excretion pattern in any given subject appeared to be similar from cycle to cycle" (*Rocca* and *Alber,* 1967). *Taymor* stellt dagegen aufgrund seiner Untersuchung von sechs Zyklen fest: „The most consistent characteristic to be noted in the cycles studied here was the degree of variability, not only from subject to subject but from cycle to cycle in the same subject (*Taymor, Lieberman, Rizkallah,* 1969). In der Monographie von 1971 geht *Keller* aufgrund eigener Daten ausführlich auf die Pathologie der Gonadotropinsekretion und auf deren medikamentöse Beeinflussung ein.

Erst mit Hilfe der Immunoassays wurden detaillierte Einzelmessungen und Verlaufsuntersuchungen bei physiologischen und pathologischen Zuständen möglich. *Burger, Catt* und *Brown* (1968) untersuchten die Beziehung zwischen Plasma-LH und der Östrogenausscheidung. „The initial increase in urinary estrogens preceded that of LH, and in those cycles in which the day of maximum LH concentration could be defined precisely, this occured either on the same day as the midcycle peak estrogen value or 1–2 days later" (*Burger* et al., 1968).

Die tägliche individuelle Ausscheidung von Östrogenen und Pregnandiol und von Serum-FSH und LH wurde von *Goebelsmann, Midgley* und *Jaffe* (1969) untersucht. „Analysis of the daily temporal relationship between these hormones revealed a peak of urinary E2 on the day preceding the peak of LH and FSH at midcycle in all 5 subjects. . . . Pregnanediol excretion also appeared to rise on the day preceding the LH and FSH peak, reaching luteal phase values 2–3 days following the gonadotropin peak. The data are consistent with the hypothesis that elaboration of estradiol, and possibly progesterone, by the maturing follicle may elicit the surge of both LH and FSH at midcycle" (*Goebelsmann* et al., 1969). *Johansson* und *Wide* (1969) fanden keine ansteigenden Progesteronwerte vor dem LH-Peak. „The maximal LH peak levels lasted for 16–20 h at which time the plasma progesterone rose to a concentration of 1–2 ng / ml. Following the fall in the LH concentration, there was a rapid rise in the plasma progesterone concentration, indicating the formation of a corpus luteum. The lowest basal body temperature coincided with the first significant rise in LH levels" (*Johansson* and *Wide,* 1969).

Strott, Yoshimi, Ross und *Lipsett* konnten zeigen, daß 17-hydroxyprogesteron zusammen mit dem LH-Anstieg zunimmt. „Our findings suggest that 17-hydroxyprogesterone can serve as an index of follicular maturation as well as of corpus luteum function, whereas progesterone reflects corpus luteum activity only" (*Strott* et al., 1969). *Abraham, Odell, Swerdloff* und *Hopper* fanden in allen normalen Zyklen einen mittzyklischen E2- und 17-OHP-Peak. „At the present time, a cause-to-effect relationship between these steroids and the ovulatory surge of gonadotropins cannot be ascertained" (*Abraham* et al., 1971). *Johansson, Wide* und *Gemzell* wiesen darauf hin, daß die Variationen der hormonellen Veränderungen zwischen verschiedenen Zyklen der gleichen Frau geringer sind, als die zwischen Zyklen verschiedener Frauen (*Johansson* et al., 1971).

Die Sensitivität und Prezision der RIAs erlaubte Verlaufskontrollen in kurzen Abständen. *Thomas, Walkiers* und *Ferin* (1970) beobachteten einen biphasischen LH-Peak. *Midgley* und *Jaffe* bestimmten LH in stündlichen Abständen. „The sampling was to long to permit an exact determination of the frequency of the peaks which appeared to occur at approximately 2 $\frac{1}{2}$ hour intervals. The largest LH excursions were noted during the ascending and descending phases of the major LH peak at midcycle and during the luteal phase of the cycle. These obvservations are compatible with the hypothesis that serum concentrations of LH, and possibly FSH, are maintained by brief periods of release followed by periods of little or no release" (*Midgley* and *Jaffe,* 1971).

1966 erschienen die Publikationen von *W. D. Odell, G. T. Ross* und *P. L. Rayford,* von *A. R. Midgley,* von *K. D. Bagshawe, C. E. Wilde* und *A. H. Orr,* von *P. Franchimont,* sowie von *L. Wide* und *J. Porath. Paul Franchimont* (˙1934 Liége – † 1994 Liége) wies bei postmenopausalen Frauen neben den erhöhten FSH- und LH-Spiegeln eine episodische Fluktuation der Gonadotropine und auch von GnRH nach (*Franchimont,* 1967).

Kurzfristig wiederholte Messungen ergaben bei Ratten (*Gay* et al., 1969) und bei Affen (*Dierschke* et al., 1970) Oszillationen in regelmäßigen Abständen. Im Ovarialzyklus der Frau sind Frequenz und Amplitude der Pulse Zyklus-abhängig (*Yen* et al., 1972). *Ernst Knobil* (˙1926 Berlin) im Department of Physiology in Pittsburgh zeigte beim Rhesusaffen, daß die pulsatile Verabreichung von LHRH in Abständen von ein bis zwei Stunden zur normalen Gonadenfunktion führt, dagegen die kontinuierliche zu einer Suppression der Gonadotropine (*Dierschke* et al., 1970, *Knobil,* 1973, 1974, 1980).

Regulation of Human Gonadotropins:
X. Episodic Fluctuation of LH During the Menstrual Cycle[1]

A. R. MIDGLEY, Jr.,[2] AND ROBERT B. JAFFE

Reproductive Endocrinology Program, Department of Pathology and Department of Obstetrics and Gynecology, The University of Michigan, Ann Arbor, Michigan 48104

ABSTRACT. Serum concentrations of LH and FSH in 49 samples obtained at consecutive hourly intervals from seven women at different phases of the menstrual cycle have been determined by radioimmunoassay. In all cases, hourly analysis indicated that serum concentrations of LH, and possibly FSH, are maintained as a series of peaks of variable magnitude. The sampling interval was too long to permit an exact determination of the frequency of the peaks which appeared to occur at approximately 2½ hour intervals. The largest LH excursions were noted during the ascending and descending phases of the major LH peak at midcycle and during the luteal phase of the cycle. These observations are compatible with the hypothesis that serum concentrations of LH, and possibly FSH, are maintained by brief periods of release followed by periods of little or no release. (*J Clin Endocr* **33**: 962, 1971)

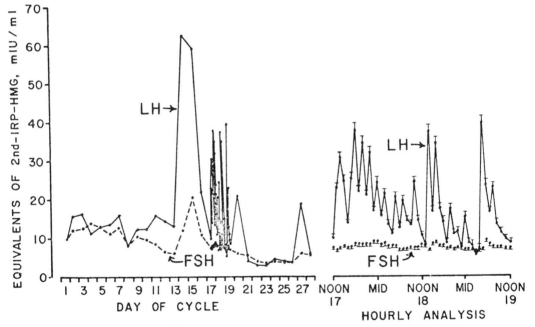

FIG. 1. Concentrations of LH and FSH in serum obtained daily from a subject with a 28 day menstrual cycle. The major surge in LH occurring at midcycle was observed on day 14. On days 17–19, 49 consecutive hourly samples of serum were obtained and analyzed. The results of these latter samples are shown on the portion of the figure to the right on an expanded time scale. The vertical bars represent one standard error of the mean of duplicate estimates as determined with the radioimmunoassay analysis program described in the text. Note that marked fluctuation in LH concentration can be observed during this period while the concentrations of FSH remain relatively stable.

Midgley, A. R., R. B. Jaffe: Regulation of Human Gonadotropins: X. Episodic fluctuation of LH during the menstruell cycle. (© Endocrine Society). J. Clin. Endocrinol. 33 (1971) 962–969.

Besonderes Interesse fanden die Veränderungen der Hypophysenfunktion in der Kindheit und Pubertät. *P. S. Brown* untersuchte die Gonadotropinausscheidung in der Pubertät. „In normal girls before puberty the excretion of FSH is high and of ICSH is low, ICSH increasing as puberty progesses. This normal pattern is reflected in the results from abnormal subjects. … There is, therefore, a constancy of pattern throughout the results from the girls, and the results from the boys are clearly contrasted. They show no evidence of a progessive increase in ICSH excretion as puberty progresses nor of a relative deficiency when puberty is delayed" (*B. S. Brown,* 1958). In einer umfangreichen Studie mit 459 Urinproben von 44 Kindern im Alter von vier bis zehn Jahren konnten *Kulin* et al. Gesamtgonadotropinaktivität mit dem Maus-Uterus Test nachweisen. Die Autoren betonen, daß eine Einzelbestimmung nicht repräsentativ ist für den endokrinen Status (*Kulin* et al., 1967). In den gleichen Urinproben wurde mit RIAs FSH und LH bestimmt. „The increase of LH was gradual; FSH excretion doubled between ages 5−6 and 7−8. No significant differences in the excretion of LH or FSH between boys and girls appeared until the age group 9−10, when LH was significantly higher in boys, and FSH was higher in girls. There were no marked increases in urinary LH excretion just prior to, or coincident with, the appearance of the earliest physical changes of puberty. Comparison of the RIA results and the results of the mouse uterine weight assay showed that the LH content but not the FSH content of the urine was correlated with the bioassay results" (*A. B. Rifkind* et al., 1970). Im Hämagglutinationhemmtest fanden *Sciarra* und *Leone* (1970) einen altersabhängigen Anstieg von LH bei Knaben mit einer steilen Zunahme mit Beginn der Pubertät. *Faiman* und *Winter* (1971) beobachteten höhere FSH- und LH-Serum-Konzentrationen bei Mädchen im Vergleich zu Jungen. *Hayes* und *Johanson* (1972) spekulierten aufgrund ihrer FSH- und LH-Messungen bei Mädchen: „Premenarchial and early postmenarchial girls have gonadotropin surges similar to adult midcycle ovulatory peaks. They presage evolution of the adult gonadotropin pattern in the subsequent postmenarchial years."

HCG wurde erstmals 1958 als Marker bei Trophoblasttumoren benutzt (*Li* et al., 1958). *Reisfeld* und *Hertz* reinigten hCG aus dem Urin von Tumorpatienten. „A comparison of some of the physical-chemical properties of the hormone obtained from the pregnancy source and from the trophoblastic source suggests a possible difference between the hormones obtained from the two sources" (*Reisfeld* u. *Hertz,* 1960). In Tumorextrakten, Plasma und Urin konnte *Judith Vaitukaitis* (1973) neben intaktem hCG-Subunits auch „altered forms of hCG" nachweisen. 1975 berichtete die gleiche Arbeitsgruppe aus dem NIH über „Evidence for altered synthesis of human chorionic gonadotropin in gestational tumors" (*Vaitukaitis* u. *Ebersole,* 1976). *Yazaki* et al. (1980) fanden im Serum von Tumorpatienten drei zusätzliche Peaks in der Isoelektro-Fokussierung. In einer Vielzahl von Tumormanifestationen wurde hCG nachgewiesen: Hodentumoren (*Hobson,* 1965), Hepatom (*Floyd* und *Cohn,* 1972), Lungen-, Pankreas- und Colon-Karzinom (*Odell* et al., 1967, *Braunstein* et al., 1973, *Vaitukaitis* et al., 1976), Nebennierenrinden-Karzinom (*Gadner* et al., 1974) und in mastopathischen Zysten (*Opri* et al., 1979). Schließlich wurde hCG auch in normalem Gewebe gefunden: Testes (*Braunstein* et al., 1975), Hypophyse und Urin bei Klinefelterpatienten (*Chen* et al., 1976), Leber und Colon (*Yoshimoto* et al., 1977). Mit Hilfe des Radioreceptorassay und β-Ketten RIA für hCG konnte die Arbeitsgruppe von *Odell* hCG-artiges Material in allen Geweben nachweisen. „We hypothesize: 1. That this hCG-like material in normal tissues has the protein structure of hCG but does not possess the carbohydrate moieties of placental hCG and probably has little or no bioactivity in vivo and 2. that the trophoblastic cell is not unique in its ability to synthesize hCG but has developed the ability to glycosylate hCG, transforming a ubiquitous cellular protein in a hormone, hCG might better be called human cellular gonadotropin" (*Yoshimoto* et al., 1979). Ektopische Produktion von Glykoprotein-Hormonen bei Tumorerkrankungen wurde beschrieben (*Liddle* et al., 1969, *Omenn,* 1973, *Weintraub* und *Rosen,* 1973, *Levine* u. *Metz,* 1974).

Gonadotropingehalt in Hypophysen

Bereits 1932 wurde in der Kieler Klinik von *J. A. Schockaert* und *H. Siebke* der Gehalt des menschlichen Hypophysenvorderlappen an gonadotropen Hormonen bestimmt. Testtiere waren infantile Mäuse, denen ein kalibrierter wäßriger Extrakt der Hypophysen in fünf Injektionen in zwölfstündigen Abständen injiziert wird. Nach 96 Stunden wurden die Tiere getötet. Als Parameter für das „Follikelreifungshormon" (= Prolan A) dienten große Follikel im Ovar, Turgeszierung des Uterus und Östruszeichen der Vagina; für das Luteinisierungshormon (= Prolan B) Blutpunkte oder Corpora lutea in den Ovarien. 39 Hypophysenvorderlappen wurden untersucht. Bei reifen männlichen Neugeborenen konnte keine Aktivität gefunden werden. Post partum und post abortum waren die Werte niedrig, oder nicht meßbar. „. . . fanden wir im Hypophysenvorderlappen der Frau bis zu 4000 ME. Hormon A und bis zu 1500 ME. Hormon B, im Hypophysenvorderlappen des Mannes bis zu 3000 ME. Hormon A und bis zu 1000 ME. Hormon B. Man hat den Eindruck, daß der Gehalt an Hormon B nach der Klimax größer ist als zur Zeit der Geschlechtsreife." Diese Befunde stimmten überein mit den Ergebnissen von *K. Ehrhardt* und *B. T. Mayes* (1930) sowie von *P. Wirz* (1933). *Paul Wirz* an der Frauenklinik in Köln untersuchte sowohl die Ausscheidung von Hypophysenvorderlappenhormon als auch den Hormongehalt in Hypophysen. Hierzu wurden Vorderlappen oder ganze Hypophysen Tieren in die Rücken- oder Oberschenkelmuskulatur implantiert. Die Bestimmung im Harn erfolgte nach alkoholischer Fällung und wäßriger Extraktion des Präzipitats. Für den Hormonnachweis dienten die drei charakteristischen Reaktionen nach *Aschheim* und *Zondek*. „Wenn aber die Ovarialfunktion ohne Hypophysenvorderlappenhormone unmöglich ist, dann sind, wenigstens theoretisch, Amenorrhöen denkbar, die durch Funktionsstörungen des Hypophysenvorderlappens hervorgerufen werden. Gibt es nun tatsächlich Zeitperioden, in denen die Hypophyse ihre Sexualhormone nicht besitzt?"

1. Ich konnte in der Hypophyse von Feten, Neugeborenen und Kindern bis zum 5. Lebensjahr nur das Follikelreifungshormon nachweisen.

2. In der Mehrzahl dieser Fälle enthielt die ganze Hypophyse noch nicht eine Mäuseeinheit Hypophysenvorderlappenhormon A (H.V.H. A); der Vorderlappen dürfte etwa vom 1. Lebensjahr an das Hormon in dieser Menge besitzen.

3. Das H.V.H. A wird im Harn von Kindern, wenn überhaupt, nur in sehr geringen Mengen ausgeschieden.

4. Es wird deshalb angenommen, daß das H.V.H. A das Follikelwachstum in den kindlichen Ovarien fördert.

5. Das Luteinisierungshormon wird erst später in der Hypophyse nachweisbar, wahrscheinlich erst kurze Zeit vor der Geschlechtsreife.

6. Dieser Befund weist daraufhin, daß die Produktion des H.V.H. B in wirksamen Mengen erst in den Pubertätsjahren einsetzt.

7. Die vermehrte Produktion von H.V.H. A und die Aufnahme der Produktion von H.V.H. B durch die Hypophyse zur Zeit der Geschlechtsreife sind diejenigen Kräfte, die den Beginn des ovariellen Zyklus auslösen.

8. Die Ursache für die ruhende Ovarialtätigkeit im Kindesalter liegt vornehmlich in der Hypophyse und weniger in den Ovarien, zumal im Tierexperiment durch genügende Zufuhr von H.V.H. Follikelreifung und Luteinisierung in infantilen Ovarien erzeugt werden können."

Bei der Untersuchung von Schwangeren und Wöchnerinnen ergaben sich folgende Befunde:

1. „In den Hypophysen von Wöchnerinnen sind in den ersten Tagen nach der Entbindung keine Sexualhormone nachweisbar.

2. Der Zeitpunkt, zu dem die H.V.H. wieder nachweisbar werden, ist verschieden und scheint abhängig zu sein von der Schwangerschaftsdauer.

3. Wenn die Schwangerschaft in frühen Monaten unterbrochen wird, so scheinen die H.V.H. in der Hypophyse früher nachweisbar zu werden.

4. Nach ausgetragener Schwangerschaft ist das H.V.H. A oft erst zwei bis drei Wochen H.V.H. B wahrscheinlich vier Wochen, sicher aber fünf Wochen nach der Entbindung in der Hypophyse wieder vorhanden.

5. Zu der Zeit, wo das H.V.H. post partum erstmalig in der Hypophyse wieder nachweisbar wird, findet die erste Ovulation statt."

„Bei 13 amenorrhoischen Frauen wurde die H.V.H.-Ausscheidung gemessen.

1. „Das H.V.H. A wird nur bei den schweren Formen von Amenorrhö vermehrt im Harn ausgeschieden und zwar in gleichen Mengen wie im Harn operativ kastrierter Frauen kurze Zeit nach dem Eingriff.
2. Wenn das H.V.H. A in Mengen von 110 M.E. im Harn vorhanden war, konnte ich das Follikulin im Harn mit der Methode von *Frank* und *Goldberger* nicht nachweisen.
3. Wenn das Hormon des Follikels im Harn wieder nachweisbar wurde, war der Gehalt des Harns an H.V.H. A niedriger als vorher.
4. Ich konnte das H.V.H. A in fünffach konzentrierten Harnextrakten nicht nachweisen, wenn Follikulin in Mengen von 10 und 35 M.E. im Harn enthalten war.
5. Die Befunde sprechen dafür, daß der Gehalt des Harns an H.V.H. A bei einer Amenorrhö abhängig ist von der noch vorhandenen Follikeltätigkeit."

Abschließend stellt *Wirz* fest: „Es gibt Zeitperioden, in denen das Fehlen des Zyklus wohl in erster Linie zurückzuführen ist auf eine verminderte Produktion des Vorderlappens, z.B. vor der Pubertät und unmittelbar nach der Schwangerschaft. Es gibt andere Zeitperioden, in denen die Sexualdrüsen selbst eine verminderte oder sogar aufgehobene Follikeltätigkeit besitzen, trotzdem die übergeordneten Sexualhormone in hinreichender Menge gebildet werden. Hier scheint nicht alleine die Ausscheidung der H.V.H. von dem Funktionszustand der Ovarien abhängig zu sein, sondern sogar die Produktion. Das würde aber bedeuten, daß die Produktionsleistung der ‚übergeordneten' Sexualdrüse wieder abhängig ist von der Funktion der eigentlichen Sexualdrüse" (*P. Wirz*, 1933). *C. Pfeiffer* im Zoological Laboratory bei *Emil Witschi* in Iowa untersuchte Geschlechtsunterschiede der Hypophyse und deren Abhängigkeit von den Gonaden. „The hypophysis in the rat at birth is bipotential and capable of beeing differentiated as either male or female, depending upon whether an ovary or a testis is present. The hypophysis of the male, whether normal or castrated and with its testes reimplanted ectopically, releases only follicle stimulator. The hypophysis of the female releases both follicle stimulator and luteinizer. ... These experiments prove that the sex difference in the hypophysis is not genetic but is secondary and dependent upon the presence of differentiated sex glands" (*Pfeiffer*, 1936).

Der Gonadotropingehalt in Hypophysen von zwei Frauen wurde von *R. C. Bahn* et al. 1953 gemessen. „The pituitary gland of the adult human female contains equal activity of FSH and LH. Urine from the adult female, however, contains more FSH activity than LH activity." *M. E. Simpson* et al. (1956) untersuchten 1956 den Hormongehalt von Hypophysen bei Macaca mulatta. „Individual anterior pituitaries as well as pooled glands of Macaca mulatta have been assayed in hypophysectomized immature female rats for their content of trophic hormones, particular gonadotrophic hormones.

1. In the adult female macaque, the content of follicle stimulating hormone was highest between the ninth and eleventh day of the cycle. The content of interstitial hormone was also maximum at this time of the cycle. The ratio of ICSH to FSH was highest (10 to 1) on days eleven and 15.

2. In adult male anterior pituitary the total content of ICSH and FSH and the ratio between these hormones was approximately the same as in the adult female pituitaries at beginning and end of menstrual cycle. The gonadotrophic hormone content of pituitaries of immature animals was lower than in adults.

3. Other trophic hormones in the adult female pituitary, thyrotrophic, adrenocorticotrophic and growth hormones, did not change in amount during the menstrual cycle" (*Simpson, van Wagenen, Carter,* 1956).

A. R. Currie und *J. B. Dekanski* (1961) in den Organon Laboratories in Newhouse, Schottland fanden, daß der in Salzlösung extrahierte Gehalt an Gonadotropin mit zunehmendem Alter bei beiden Geschlechtern ansteigt. Als Assay wurde das Ovargewicht und die vaginale Verhornung bei immaturen Ratten, sowie das Prostatagewicht bei hypophysektomierten Ratten benutzt. Das FSH : ICSH-Verhältnis bei Männern über 50 war eins zu eins.

Mit Hilfe des OAAD-Tests bestimmte *R. J. Ryan* den LH-Gehalt in Einzelhypophysen von 19 Männern, 16 Frauen und vier Kindern. Sowohl der spezifische (pro Gewichtseinheit) als auch der Gesamtgehalt pro Hypophyse nahm mit dem Alter bei beiden Geschlechtern zu (1961). *Elrick* und Mitarbeiter (1964) fanden, daß fixierte (embalmed) Hypophysen eine gute Quelle zur Gewinnung von tropen Hormonen ist. Die Aktivität von FSH, LH, GH, und TSH war geringer als in frischen Organen, die Prolaktin- und ACTH-Aktivität dagegen leicht größer.

Bei der Extraktion humaner Hypophysen zur Gewinnung von Gonadotropin zur klinischen Anwendung, ergab sich die Möglichkeit den Gehalt von Einzeldrüsen an hormoneller Aktivität zu messen. Auf dem 3. annual meeting des Europian Pediatric Endocrinology Club in Hamburg 1965 wurde berichtet, daß die Aktivität pro Hypophyse 15- bis 20mal größer ist, als die tägliche Ausscheidung. Im Pool von 1000 Drüsen, meist von älteren

Menschen, wurden im Mittel 1000 hMG-Einheiten pro Hypophyse gemessen. Bei Feten wurden zwei bis sechs Einheiten gefunden, die gleiche Aktivität auch bei Schwangeren (*Bettendorf,* 1965). Im weiteren wurden Hypophysen von jüngeren Frauen gesammelt, um die Veränderungen im Zyklus zu untersuchen.

In 35 Einzelhypophysen akut verstorbener Frauen wurde FSH mit dem Augmentationstest und LH mit dem OAAD-Test gemessen (*Bettendorf* et al., 1969). Die Korrelation zum Zykluszeitpunkt erfolgte durch die histologische Beurteilung des Funktionszustands von Ovarien und Endometrium. Die FSH-Aktivität war im wesentlichen gleichbleibend während des Zyklus mit einem nicht signifikanten präovulatorischen Anstieg. Bei der LH-Aktivität waren die Werte zu Anfang des Zyklus hoch, fielen in der Follikelphase ab, zeigten präovulatorisch einen Anstieg und waren in der Lutealphase wieder niedrig. Bei Männern lag die Aktivität im gleichen Bereich, bei Schwangeren fand sich dagegen eine wesentlich geringere Aktivität.

De La Lastra und *Llados* (1977) machten die gleiche Beobachtung mit Hilfe eines spezifischen RIA. „The LH content was significantly lower in pregnant and post-abortion patients than in non-pregnant women. In pregnant women the lowest values were observed towards the end of gestation."

Philipp hatte bereits 1930 gonadotrope Aktivität in fetalen Drüsen nachgewiesen. In je acht Hypophysen von weiblichen und männlichen Totgeborenen im 6.–7. Monat der Schwangerschaft konnten *B. F. Rice, R. Ponthier* und *Sternberg* (1968) im Prostatalappentest LH- und im Tibiatest GH-Aktivität nachweisen. *Franchimont* und *Pasteels* (1972) zeigten, daß fetale Hypophysenkulturen in vitro etwa 200mal mehr α-subunit als intaktes LH und FSH sezernieren und nur geringe Mengen β-subunit.

„Immunoreactive pituitary FSH and LH reach their highest concentration by mid-gestation, whereas serum FSH and LH attain concentrations in the postmenopausal range at midgestation with a decrease to undetectable levels at term. Significantly higher levels of pituitary and serum FSH and LH are present in the female than in the male fetus" (*Kaplan* und *Grumbach,* 1976). Die gleichen Autoren untersuchten die Konzentration von α- und β-subunits in fetalen Hypophysen (*Kaplan* et al., 1976). Die α-subunit war im Serum und in den Hypophysen nachweisbar; dagegen nur wenig oder gar keine β-subunit. Im Gegensatz zum intakten LH und FSH fand sich kein Geschlechtsunterschied bei der α-subunit.

Aus den Untersuchungen von *Hagen* und *McNeilly* geht hervor: „The free α-subunit: LH ratio reached a peak between 10 and 14 weeks of gestation and decreases to adult ratios by term. No FSH was detected in pituitary

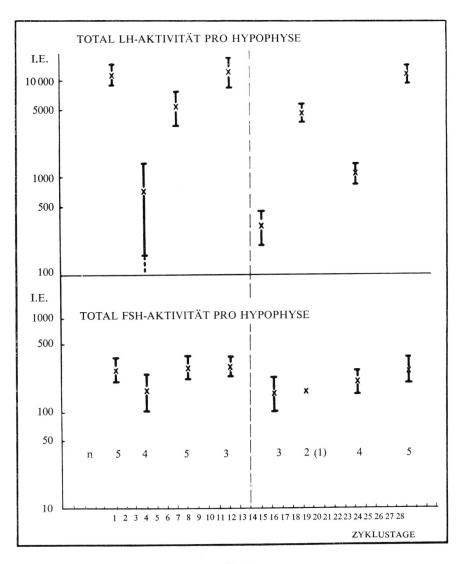

Abb. 8
FSH- und LH-Aktivität pro Hypophyse zu verschiedenen Zeiten des ovariellen Zyklus.

Bettendorf, G.: FSH- und LH-Aktivität pro Hypophyse zu verschiedenen Zeiten des Zyklus. In Louwrens, B.: Menschliche Gonadotropine. Rundtischgespräch im Tel-Hashomer Hospital, Israel, 28. Mai 1968. Acta Endocrinol. Suppl. 148, 1970 (19).

extracts from 9,5–12,5 weeks while FSH was detectable in all foetal pituitaries at term. No significant sex differences in intact hormone or subunit concentrations in the pituitary was seen. In contrast to these results the pituitary
of an anencephalic foetus (36 week of gestation) contained mainly free α-
subunit. During early gestation foetal blood levels of LH-hCG, FSH and
free α-subunit were significantly higher than at term. ... These results suggest that during foetal development the first gonadotrophin substance syn-
thetized in the foetal pituitary is the common α-subunit. Under hypopthala-
mic influence the synthesis of the β-subunit then takes place leading to the
production of the intact gonadotrophins" (*Hagen* und *McNeilly*, 1977).

Im Rahmen der Untersuchungen zur Mikroheterogenität von hypophysärem FSH untersuchte *Wide* (1989) „FSH in extracts of the anterior lobe of
pituitaries, collected at autopsy from 13 boys, 21 girls, 17 men and 26
women, measured in terms of biological activity in vitro by the Sertoli cell
aromatase bioassay, and in terms of immunological activity by a radioimmunoassay. The highest concentration of FSH in the anterior lobe found by
bioassay was in young girls, who had a mean value three to seven times higher than that in young and elderly men and women and nine times higher
than in young boys. The total amount of FSH in the pituitary found by bioassay and immunoassay was very much less in young boys than in all other
groups. The B/I ratio of FSH was higher for all the 27 children below 10
years of age than for any of the 43 adults. This difference in B/I ratio of
FSH in whole pituitary extracts persisted in fractions after electrophoretic separation. The mean B/I ratio for young girls was 1.26 times higher than
that for young boys and 2.25 times higher than that for adults. Young and
elderly men and women, had almost identical B/I ratios. All extracts were
analysed after electrophoresis and the median charge homogeneity of FSH
were estimated. The number of different forms of FSH in pituitary extracts
from a child was at least 20–30, similar to that in adult. In girls, the median
charge of FSH was similar to that of young women and significantly less negative than in elderly women. The median charge of FSH in boys was more
negative than in girls, but less negative than in both young and elderly men.
After treatment of pituitary extracts with neuraminidase, the median charge
of FSH in infants was significantly more negative than in adults. This, together with the differences in B/I ratios between children and adults, indicates a change at puberty in the molecular structure of FSH from juvenile to
adult forms of the hormone (*Wide*, 1989).

Eine Hypersekretion von LH und FSH bei einem Mann mit einem Hypophysenadenom wurde von *Snyder* und *Sterling* berichtet. Die Werte normalisierten sich nach Hypophysektomie (*Snyder* und *Sterling*, 1976).

Gonadotropinaktivität wurde bei zahlreichen Spezies nachgewiesen. *Otsuka* beschrieb 1956 FSH und LH in Lachs-Hypophysen. *Donaldson* et al. (1972) fanden ein Gonadotropin in Lachs-Hypophysen, das für die testikuläre Entwicklung verantwortlich ist. Mit ethanolischem Ammoniumacetatpuffer konnte ein Glykoprotein aus Hypophysen vom Dornhai extrahiert werden, entsprechend der Extraktion vom humanen Hypophysen (*Scanes* et al., 1972). Eine Abhängigkeit der Ovarfunktion von Hypophysenhormonen bei Fischen (*Dodd*, 1972; *Reinboth*, 1972), bei Reptilien (*Licht*, 1972) und bei Vögeln (*Meier* und *MacGregor*, 1972) wurde nachgewiesen. *Paul Licht* berichtete 1976 auf der Laurentian Hormon Conference umfassend über „Evolution of Gonadotropin Structure and Function" (*Licht* et al., 1977). FSH und LH bei Amphibien, Reptilien und Vögeln wurden untersucht und mit denen von Säugetier und Mensch verglichen.

Chemie der Gonadotropine

Erst mit der Entwicklung der Ionen-Austausch-Chromatographie und der Gelfiltration wurde eine weitgehende Aufklärung der chemischen Struktur der Gonadotropine möglich. Folgende Zusammenfassung schreibt *Morris* in einem Übersichtsartikel „Chemistry of Gonadotropins" 1955 im British Medical Journal: „It will be seen from the foregoing review that only two gonadotrophic hormones have been obtained in a satisfactory state of purity, and that even here, in both cases, there is evidence that the biological activity may reside in a small portion of the molecule or may be due to a trace constituent. In comparison with ACTH, the gonadotrophins have received relatively little attention from the chemist in the past decade and it is very desirable that they should be re-examined by more modern methods of fractionation. All the known gonadotrophins are glycoproteins, and the carbohydrate residue appears in most cases to be essential for biological activity. This fact only emphasizes our ignorance of the chemistry of glycoproteins in general and it would appear that advances in our knowledge of the structure and mode of action of the gonadotrophins must await corresponding advances in this field of protein chemistry" (*Morris*, 1955). Zehn Jahre später sind die Befunde wesentlich umfangreicher geworden, aber die chemische Struktur der Gonadotropine ist nur annäherungsweise geklärt (*Morris*, 1966).

Beim hCG wurden Präparationen mit einer biologischen Aktivität nicht über 8–9000 IU/mg erhalten (*Li*, 1949). *Got* und *Bourillon* gelang 1960 eine Anreicherung auf 12 000 IU/mg in einem homogenen Präparat aus Schwangerenurin (*Got*, 1960). Die Glycoproteinstruktur wurde beschrieben, der Kohlenhydratanteil mit 30 % bestimmt, das Molekulargewicht durch Ultrazentrifugation mit 30 000. Übereinstimmende Werte fanden *Blobel* et al. 1962 und *Nydick* et al. 1964. Präparate mit höherer biologischer Aktivität wurden aus Trophoblasttumoren gewonnen (*Reisfeld* und *Hertz*, 1960, *Wilde* und *Bagshawe*, 1965). Aus kommerziellen hCG-Präparaten resultierten schließlich biologische Aktivitäten von 12–18 000 IU/mg. (*Bahl*, 1969,

RÉCENTES ACQUISITIONS
SUR LA GONADOTROPINE CHORIALE HUMAINE

par R. Got (*)

HISTORIQUE

L A présence, dans le sang et l'urine de femme enceinte d'une substance possédant une activité gonadotrope, capable de produire une maturité précoce chez les rongeurs impubères, fut montrée par Aschheim et Zondek (2) en 1927. Les auteurs la dénommèrent « Prolan ».

1° — ORIGINE.

Quoique cette découverte servit de base à un diagnostic de grossesse, cette hormone ne fut pas distingée a priori de l'hormone hypophysaire, et une confusion régna pendant plusieurs années quant à l'origine des divers facteurs gonadotropes humains.

En effet, il fallut attendre des données expérimentales établissant que le principe gonadotrope qui apparaît durant la grossesse émane du placenta et non de l'hypophyse (16, 22).

La démonstration la plus convaincante de l'origine placentaire fut donnée par la production « in vitro » de gonadotropine dans des cultures de tissus placentaires, particulièrement de cellules de Langhans (33, 18). Des études histo-chimiques (35) et des expériences de transplantation oculaire de tissus chorioniques (25) confirmèrent cette origine.

Aussi, les anciennes appellations, « prolan de grossesse » ou « substance anté-hypophysaire-like », furentelles abandonnées au profit de la dénomination actuelle : gonadotropine choriale humaine.

(*) *Laboratoire de Chimie Biologique* (Directeur : Professeur M. F. JAYLE), *Faculté de Médecine*, 45, *rue des Saints-Pères*, *Paris-VI*.

TABLEAU I. — Schéma d'une préparation portant sur 27 litres d'urine titrant 23.000 UI/litre (621.000 UI)

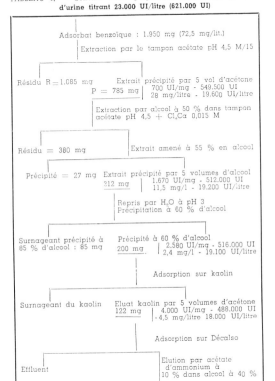

Path. Biol., 1960, *Vol.* 8, N° 17-18, 1583-1592.

Got, R.: Récentes Acquisitions sur la gonadotropine choriale humaine. Path. Biol. 8 (1960) 1583–1592.

— Nouvelles caractéristiques physico-chimiques de la gonadotropine chorionique humaine	
Activité (UI/mg)	10.000 à 12.000
N (%)	10,5
C (%)	44,2
H (%)	7,3
Taux en polypeptide (%)	57
Constante de sédimentation, S_{20} (cm. sec⁻¹ dyne⁻¹)	$2,7 \times 10^{-13}$
Constante de diffusion, D_{20} (cm² sec⁻¹)	$8,2 \times 10^{-7}$
Volume spécifique partiel (ml/g)	0,727
Poids moléculaire (formule de Svedberg)	30.000
— (diffusion de la lumière)	29.000
Rapport de friction	1,28
Mobilité électrophorétique, pH 8,6 $\mu = 0,1$ (cm² sec⁻¹ volt⁻¹)	$2,5 \times 10^{-5}$
Point iso-électrique	2,95
du/dpH₀	$1,05 \times 10^{-5}$
E $\dfrac{1\%}{1\ cm}$	4,25
M tyrosine/M tryptophane	2,4
Pouvoir rotatoire [α]D	— 68°
Résidu NH₂-terminal	Néant
Résidu COOH-terminal	Glycocolle
Hexoses (%)	11
Mannose/Galactose	1
Fucose (%)	1,2
Hexosamines (%)	8,7
Glucosamine/Galactosamine	4
Hexoses/Hexosamines	1,26
Acides sialiques (%)	8,5
Action folliculo-stimulante	Néant
Action corticotrope	Néant
Stimulation des cellules interstitielles	+++

Got, R.: Récentes Acquisitions sur la gonadotropine choriale humaine. Path. Biol. 8 (1960) 1583–1592.

van Hell et al., 1968, *Canfield* et al., 1971, *Gräßlin* et al., 1970, *Merz* et al., 1974).

1. „An hCG preparation of a biological potency of 18 800 (16 200–21 800) iu / mg was isolated.

2. Immunochemically homogenous hCG appeared to consist of one to six components all carrying biological activity.

3. The biological potencies of hCG preparations increase in the same order as their NANA contents and the electrophoretic mobilities of their components.

4. It is not clear whether these components originate as such from the chorion or whether less potent molecules are degradation products of the biologically most active one.

5. The structural requirements for the biological and for the immuno-chemical activities are not identical" (*van Hell* et al., 1966).

Bahl gelang die Dissoziation von intaktem hCG in subunits (*Bahl,* 1969), die Gelelektrophorese in Polyacrylamid ergab zwei Banden (*Canfield* et al., 1970). Die Aufklärung der nicht-kovalenten Bindung der subunits erfolgte durch *Swaminathan* und *Bahl* (1970) und wurde ein Jahr später von *Morgan* und *Canfield* (1971) bestätigt. Die Isoelektrofokussierung ergab einen Polymorphismus von hCG und den subunits (*Bahl,* 1969, *van Hell,* 1968, *Gräßlin et al., 1972, Merz* et al., 1974). Die biologischen Aktivitäten der po-

Nature of the Subunits of Human Chorionic Gonadotropin

FRANCIS J. MORGAN[1] AND ROBERT E. CANFIELD[2]

Department of Medicine and The International Institute for the Study of Human Reproduction, College of Physicians and Surgeons, Columbia University, New York, New York 10032

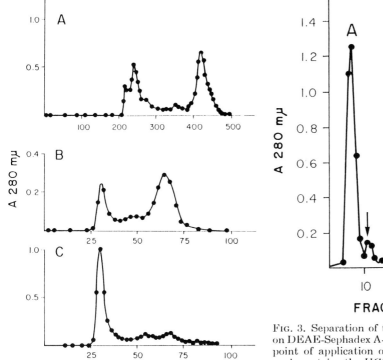

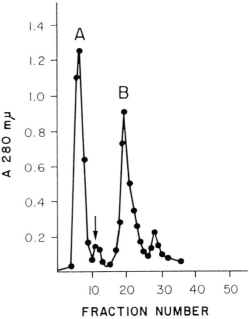

FIG. 3. Separation of the subunits of native HCG on DEAE-Sephadex A-25. The arrow represents the point of application of the second buffer. The A peak contains the HCG-α subunit and the B peak the HCG-β subunit. For further details, see text.

FIG. 2. A: Chromatography of urea-dissociated SCM-HCG on Sephadex G-25; B: rechromatography of the first peak from Fig. 2A (200–275 ml) on Sephadex G-100. The second peak contains the SCM-HCG-α subunit and the first some contaminating SCM-HCG-β subunit. C: Rechromatography of the second peak of Fig. 2A (375–475 ml) on Sephadex G-100. The peak contains SCM-HCG-β subunit. Details of the chromatography are given in the text.

Morgan, F. J., R. E. Canfield: Nature of the subunits of human chorionic gonadotropin. Endocrinology 88 (1971) 1045–1051 (© Endocrine Society).

SEPARATION OF PURIFIED HUMAN CHORIONIC GONADOTROPIN INTO SINGLE BANDS BY ISOELECTRIC FOCUSING AND THEIR CHARACTERIZATION*

R. BROSSMER, W.E. MERZ and U. HILGENFELDT

Institut für Biochemie (Med. Fak.) der Universität, Heidelberg, Germany

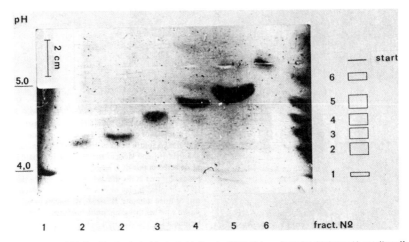

Fig. 1. Refocusing of 6 isolated bands, obtained by isoelectric focusing (right side) on a Sephadex thin layer with a gradient pH 3–10.

Brosmer, R., W. E. Merz, U. Hilgenfeldt: Separation of purified human chorionic gonadotropin into single bands by isoelectric focusing and their characterization. FEBS Letters 18 (1971) 113–115 (reprinted with kind permission from Elsevier Science, NL Sara Burgerhartstraat 25, 1055 KV Amsterdam, The Netherlands).

lymorphen Formen war nicht einheitlich (*Brossmer*, 1971, *Gräßlin*, 1972). Die Aminosäuresequenz wurde von *Bahl* et al., (1972) und *Morgan* et al., (1973) bestimmt und führte zu weitgehend gleichen Ergebnissen: β-hCG bei *Bahl* 147, bei *Morgan* 145 Aminosäuren. Der Kohlenhydratanteil liegt bei 30 % (*Got*, 1965, *Bahl*, 1969).

Griff Ross befaßte sich in einem Vortrag auf der 100. Tagung der American Gynecologic Society 1977 in Arizona mit der „Clinical relevance of research on the structure of human chorionic gonadotropin" (*Ross*, 1978).

Die Untersuchungen zur Reinigung und physiko-chemischen Charakterisierung der hypophysären Gonadotropine erfolgten im wesentlichen in folgenden Arbeitsgruppen: *Choh Hao Li, Phil G. Squire, Harold Papkoff* in Berkeley; *Sanford L. Steelman, Albert Segaloff* in New Orleans; *Alfred E. Wilhelmi, Leo E. Reichert, Albert F. Parlow* in Atlanta; *Jutisz* in Paris; *Wilfried R. Butt, Arthur C. Crooke* in Birmingham.

1949 haben *Virgil L. Koenig* und *Elmer King* in den Amour Laboratories in Chicago die Extraktion von Hypophysen mit 40 % ethanolischem Azetatpuffer beschrieben. Mit dieser Methode konnte ein Präparat zur klinischen Anwendung gewonnen werden, hHG mit FSH und LH-Aktivität (*Bettendorf* et al., 1962). Durch schrittweise Elution mit Ammoniumsulfat gelang eine Anreicherung der LH-Aktivität (*Breckwoldt* et al., 1967). *Squire* und *Li* benutzten die Ammonium-Sulfat-Fraktionierung (1958). Mit Hilfe der Zonen-Elektrophorese fand *Jutisz* 1957 fünf aktive Komponenten des gereinigten LH (*Jutisz* und *Squire*, 1958). *Squire* und *Li* gelang die Isolierung von LH auf Schafs-Hypophysen mit einem Molekulargewicht von 30 000 (*Squire* und *Li*, 1959). Eine 15 fache Anreicherung von FSH aus humanen Hypophysen mit einer Ammoniumsulfat-Fraktionierung und Reinigung an Amberlite erzielte *Li* (1958). LH aus humanen Hypophysen zeigte deutliche Unterschiede sowohl im biologischen Test, als auch physiko-chemisch (*Li* et al., 1960, *Li*, 1960). *Ute Gröschel* und *Li* bestimmten den Kohlenhydratanteil und fanden zum erstenmal Sialinsäure in hypophysärem Gonadotropin (*Gröschel* und *Li*, 1960). *Steelman* und Mitarbeiter (1959) erzielten eine Trennung von FSH und LH durch Säulenchromatographie an Carboxymethyl-Cellulose. *Squire* benutzte die Methode zur Reinigung von ICSH und erhielt ein Präparat mit hoher Aktivität und einem Molekulargewicht von 26 000 (*Squire* et al., 1962).

Butt et al. (1961) erzielten eine gute Anreicherung von FSH- und LH-Aktivität durch Carboxymethyl- und Diethylaminoethyl-Cellulose. Aminosäure und Kohlenhydratanalysen wurden von dieser Gruppe 1969 berichtet (*Barker* et al., 1969).

Das Konzept des Polymorphismus der Gonadotropine und der Existenz von Isohormonen sollte die weitere chemische Abklärung erschweren. *Li* und *Starman* fanden 1964 nach Ultrazentrifugation bei niedrigem pH zwei Produkte mit einem Molekulargewicht von 15–16 000. Sie vermuteten, daß es sich um Dimere handelte (*Li* und *Starman*, 1964). Drei Jahre später zeigte *Ward*, daß die beiden Produkte nicht identisch sind und diskutierten, daß die Gonadotropine aus zwei nicht identischen, nicht covalent gebundenen Ketten bestehen (*Ward* et al., 1967). Die Behandlung von ovinem LH mit Harnstoff bei pH 4 führte zur Dissoziation in zwei Subunits und zum Verlust der Aktivität (*De la Llosa* et al., 1967). *Papkoff* und *Samy* (1967) kamen zum gleichen Ergebnis. Die Inkubation der Subunit-Lösung ergab eine Regeneration der biologischen Aktivität. Die α- und β-Nomenklatur wurde 1970 von *Papkoff* und *Pierce* vorgeschlagen (*Papkoff*, 1995). Die Aminosäure-Sequenz für die Subunits von bovinem LH (*Pierce* et al., 1971) und

Reprinted from *Ciba Foundation Colloquia* on
Endocrinology, 13, 1960, pp. 46–64

STUDIES ON HUMAN PITUITARY GROWTH
AND GONADOTROPIC HORMONES

Choh Hao Li

Hormone Research Laboratory, University of California, Berkeley

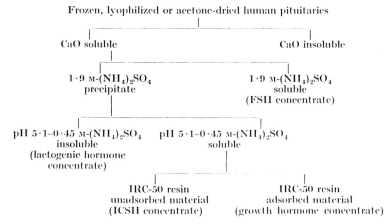

FIG. 1. A scheme for the purification of human pituitary hormone concentrates.

Li, Ch. H.: Studies on human pituitary growth and gonadotropic hormones. Ciba Coll. on Endocrinology 13 (1960) 46–64 (with permission of Churchill Livingstone).

Purification of human pituitary follicle-stimulating hormone (With Ute Gröschel)

Table VII

YIELD AND POTENCY OF FRACTIONS OBTAINED FROM
PURIFICATION PROCEDURE OF HUMAN FSH

Fraction	Weight	Procedure	Activity
	mg.		units/mg.
A	10,000	Lyophilized whole gland	
SII	250	(NH$_4$)$_2$SO$_4$ fractionation	9
G	60	Column electrophoresis	30
H	25	DEAE-cellulose chromatography	100

biological activity can be achieved with the FSH fraction SII used as starting material. An average yield of 25 mg. of highly purified FSH (fraction H) can be obtained from 10 g. of lyophilized human pituitaries; this preparation appeared

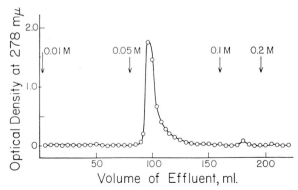

FIG. 7. Chromatography of human FSH fraction H (42 mg.) on DEAE-cellulose, equilibrated with 0·01 M-K$_2$HPO$_4$.

Li, Ch. H.: Studies on human pituitary growth and gonadotropic hormones. Ciba Coll. on Endocrinology 13 (1960) 46–64 (with permission of Churchill Livingstone).

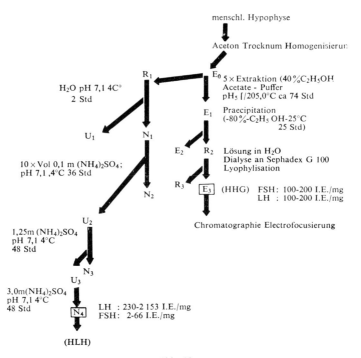

menschl. Hypophyse

Aceton Trocknum Homogenisierun

R_1 E_0 5 × Extraktion (40%C_2H_5OH
H_2O pH 7,1 4C°   Acetate - Puffer
2 Std   pH$_5$ [/205,0°C ca 74 Std

                E_1 Praecipitation
                      (-80%-C_2H_5 OH-25°C
                              25 Std)

U_1 N_1

        E_2 R_2 Lösung in H_2O
10 × Vol 0,1 m $(NH_4)_2SO_4$;   Dialyse an Sephadex G 100
pH 7,1 ,4°C 36 Std   Lyophilisation

        R_3
            $\boxed{E_3}$ (HHG) FSH: 100-200 I.E./mg
N_2 LH : 100-200 I.E./mg

U_2
1,25m $(NH_4)_2SO_4$ Chromatographie Electrofocusierung
pH 7,1 4°C
48 Std

    N_3
U_3
3,0m$(NH_4)_2SO_4$
pH 7,1 4°C
48 Std $\boxed{N_4}$ LH : 230-2 153 I.E./mg
              FSH: 2-66 I.E./mg

(HLH)

Abb. 65
Extraktionsschema von HHG und HLH.

HHG-Aktivitäten pro mg			
E_3	FSH	LH	FSH/LH
IE	100–200	100–1000	0,05–5,2
NIH	10–25 (S_1)	0,1–0,3 (B_1)	—
N_4	FSH	LH	FSH/LH
IE*	2–66	230–2153	0,01–0,06
NIH	0,1–2,5 (S_3)	0,23–1,4 (B_3)	—

Abb. 66
Übersicht der FSH- und LH-Aktivitäten und der FSH/LH-Quotienten gefunden in den
verschiedenen E_3 (HHG) und N_4 (HLH) Präparaten. (s. Abb. 65).

* Berechnet nach Reichert und Parlow (1964).

Bettendorf, G., M. Breckwoldt, Ch. Neale: Extraktionsschema von HHG und HLH und FSH-
und LH-Aktivitäten. In Louwrens, B.: 1968 (103).

Purification et propriétés physico-chimiques et biologiques de l'hormone folliculo-stimulante de Mouton

par

Marian JUTISZ, Claude HERMIER, Andrée COLONGE et Robert COURRIER

(Paris)

(*Travail du Laboratoire de Morphologie Expérimentale et Endocrinologie, Collège de France, 11, place Marcelin-Berthelot, Paris-5ᵉ.*)

TABLEAU I

PURIFICATION DE LA F.S.H. DE MOUTON
(Toutes les opérations ont lieu à 4 °C sauf indications différentes)

Poudre acétonique : 1 kilogramme d'antéhypophyses de mouton
↓ Traitement au butanol anhydre
↓ Extraction par $(NH_4)_2SO_4$ 0,1 M, à pH 8, (4 l)
Surnageant I + H_2SO_4 qsp pH 5,0, 2 h
↓
Surnageant II + $(NH_4)_2SO_4$ qsp 2 M, pH 7, 18 h
↓
Surnageant III + $(NH_4)_2SO_4$ qsp 3,6 M, pH 5, 18 h
↓
Résidu S III R1 + 1,2 l H_2O + $(NH_4)_2SO_4$ qsp 1,8 M, pH 4, 2 h
↓
Surnageant S III S2 + $(NH_4)_2SO_4$ qsp 3,6 M, pH 4, 12 h
↓
Résidu S III R3 + 0,9 l H_2O + $(NH_4)_2SO_4$ qsp 1,8 M, pH 4, 2 h
↓
Surnageant S III S4 + $(NH_4)_2SO_4$ qsp 3,6 M, pH 4, 12 h
↓
Résidu S III R5 + 0,15 l H_2O + Zn(Ac)₂ qsp 0,005 M, pH 6
↓ + EtOH abs. qsp 45 %, — 5 °C,
Surnageant (Zn S45) + EtOH abs. qsp 80 %, —10 °C, 12 h
↓
Résidu Zn R 80 (650 mg, 0,6 U.N.I.H.-F.S.H.-S1)
↓
Chromatographie sur D.E.A.E.-cellulose
↓ Tampon Tris-HCl 0,008 M, pH 7,3
↓ Élution graduelle par NaCl (0,1 M)
Fraction « De » (40 mg, 5 à 10 U.N.I.H.-F.S.H.-S1)
Filtration sur Sephadex G-100
↓ Tampon acétate de pyridine 0,1 M, pH 5
Fraction « Sx » (5 à 8 mg, 25 à 30 U.N.I.H.-F.S.H.-S1)

Justiz, M., C. Hermier, A. Colonge, R. Courrier: Purification e propriétés physico-chimique et biologiques de l'hormone folliculo- stimulante de Mouton. Ann. d'Endocrinologie 26 (1965) 670–682.

von bovinem LH (*Papkoff* et al., 1971) ist seit 1971 bekannt. Geringe übereinstimmende Korrekturen erfolgten 1973 von *Papkoff* und von *Ward* auf der Laurentian Hormone Conference (*Papkoff* et al., 1973 und *Ward* et al., 1973). Die Aminosäuresequenz der Subunits von hCG wurde von *Bahl* (1972, 1973) und von *Morgan* und *Canfield* (1973) aufgeklärt. Beim Vergleich der Subunits von TSH mit denen von LH fand *Pierce,* daß eine, die α-

[Reprinted from Biochemistry, **1**, 412 (1962).]

Purification and Characterization of Human Pituitary Interstitial Cell–Stimulating Hormone*

Phil G. Squire, Choh Hao Li, and Richard N. Andersen

From the Hormone Research Laboratory, University of California, Berkeley, California

Received February 21, 1962

TABLE III

COMPARISON OF SOME PROPERTIES OF OVINE AND HUMAN ICSH

Properties	Ovine	Human
$s_{20,w}$	2.70 S	2.71 S
Molecular weight	30,000	26,000
Isoelectric point	7.3	5.4
"Leak point" IRC-50	6.2	5.6
Specific activity (units/mg)	300	1,500

Purification and properties of human ICSH (With P. G. Squire)

Table VIII

YIELD AND POTENCY OF FRACTIONS OBTAINED FROM PURIFICATION PROCEDURE OF HUMAN ICSH

Fraction	Yield	Procedure	Activity
	mg.		units/mg.
A	10,000	Lyophilized pituitaries	
U	150	IRC-50 resin unadsorbed obtained from growth hormone isolation steps	37
HA	95	pH 4·5-$(NH_4)_2SO_4$ fractionation	57
HB	33	Column electrophoresis	135
HC	5	IRC-50 resin chromatography	240

Squire, P. G., Ch. H. Li, R. N. Andersen: Purification and characterization of human pituitary interstitial cell-stimulating hormone. (© American Chemical Society) Biochemistry 1 (1962) 412–418.

Reprinted from
Biochimica et Biophysica Acta **147, 1967**
Elsevier Publishing Company
Amsterdam
Printed in The Netherlands

175

Hormone Research Laboratory, School of Medicine,
University of California Medical Center,
San Francisco, Calif. (U.S.A.)

HAROLD PAPKOFF
T. S. ANANTHA SAMY

PRELIMINARY NOTES

BBA 31015

Isolation and partial characterization of the polypeptide chains of ovine interstitial cell-stimulating hormone

AMINO ACID COMPOSITION OF THE SUB-UNITS OF OVINE ICSH

Amino acid	Ovine ICSH (μmoles/mg protein)	Sub-unit, CI (μmoles/mg protein)	Sub-unit, CII (μmoles/mg protein)
Lysine	0.372	0.593	0.171
Histidine	0.181	0.177	0.152
Arginine	0.324	0.216	0.344
Aspartic acid	0.367	0.396	0.282
Threonine	0.410	0.555	0.352
Serine	0.357	0.386	0.445
Glutamic acid	0.395	0.519	0.370
Proline	0.780	0.538	1.120
Glycine	0.312	0.287	0.412
Alanine	0.418	0.455	0.422
Cystine (half)	0.505	0.486	0.464
Valine	0.415	0.309	0.352
Methionine	0.150	0.208	0.111
Isoleucine	0.212	0.137	0.201
Leucine	0.402	0.203	0.581
Tyrosine	0.234	0.297	0.099
Phenylalanine	0.248	0.320	0.185

Papkoff, H., T. S. A. Samy: Isolation and partial characterization of the polypeptide chains of ovine interstitial cell-stimulating hormone. Biochim. Biophs. Acta 147 (1967) 175–177 (with kind permission of Elsevier Science).

subunit der beiden Hormone gleich und austauschbar war (*Pierce* et al., 1971). *Paul Franchimont* behandelte ausführlich in der Royal Society of Medicin im Juli in London die Problematik des Polymorphismus der Polypeptide Hormone (*Franchimont* et al., 1972). „It is impossible at the present time to assign a physiological significance to every cause of heterogeneity of protein and polypeptide hormones. Nevertheless, the emerging concept of prohormones for peptide hormones, either in the form of higher molecular weight precursors or in the form of lower molecular weight subunits, strongly suggests that prohormones have some function. ... Obviously many years of research will be needed before the significance and possible functions of all the causes of hormone heterogeneity can be elucidated. It

CHEMISTRY

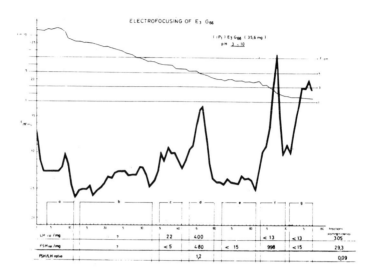

LH ı.u /mg		?		22	400		< 13	≤ 13		fractions	305
FSH ı.u /mg		?		< 5	480	< 15	998	<15			29,3
FSH/LH ratio					1,2						0,09

Fig. 6

Electrofocusing of E$_3$ pH 3 - 10

Fraction	pH	FSH		L H		FSH/LH ratio
		ı.u/mg	Fiducial limits	ı.u / mg	Fiducial limits	
Starting material E3 G66		29,3	(20 - 34,8)	305	(287 - 323)	0,09
a	10	?		?	-	
b	7.8	?		?	-	
c	6-7	<5	-	22	(10,8 - 34)	
d	5	480	(372 - 558)	,410	(400 - 420)	1,2
e	4	< 15	-		-	
f	3	998	(374 -1488)	< 13	-	
g	1,5	<15	-	< 13	-	

Table 4

Relative potencies of FSH and LH of the fractions obtained by electrofocusing

Bettendorf, G., M. Breckwoldt, P. J. Czygan, A. Fock, T. Kumasaka: Fractionation of human pituitary gonadotropins (extraction, gelfiltration and electrofocusing). In Rosemberg, E. (ed.): Gonadotropins. Geron-X Los- Altos, Calif. 1968 (13–24).

ISOLATION AND PARTIAL CHARACTERIZATION OF SEVERAL DIFFERENT CHORIONIC GONADOTROPIN (HCG) COMPONENTS

D. GRAESSLIN, H.C. WEISE and P.J. CZYGAN

Abteilung für klin. u. experimentelle Endokrinology der Universitäts-Frauenklinik, 2 Hamburg 20, Germany

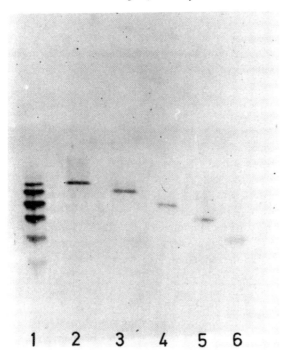

Fig. 1. Analytical gel isoelectric focusing pattern of CM fraction H_2C_3 of HCG (pos. 1) and 5 HCG components, isolated by preparative gel isoelectric focusing from H_2C_3 (pos. 2–6). 5% Polyacrylamide gel, 2% Ampholine, pH 3–6. Staining with Coomassie Brillant Blue. Anode at the top.

Graesslin, D., H. C. Weise, P. J. Czygan: Isolation and partial characterization of several different chorionic gonadotropin (HCG) components. (reprinted with kind persission of Elsevier Sciende) FEBS Letters 20 (1972) 87–89.

Polymorphism of human pituitary lutropin (LH)

Isolation and partial characterization of seven isohormones

H.C. Weise, D. Graesslin, V. Lichtenberg and G. Rinne

Abteilung für klinische und experimentelle Endokrinologie, Universitäts-Frauenklinik, Martinistr. 52, 2000 Hamburg-Eppendorf, FRG

Received 20 May 1983

The complete microheterogeneous system of human pituitary lutropin was demonstrated by gel isoelectric focusing. In addition 7 LH isohormones could be isolated by preparative column focusing and characterized with respect to physicochemical, biological and immunological properties. The in vivo biopotencies ranged from 4.50–11.50 IU/mg, the in vitro bioactivity was from 1.20–10.10 IU/mg, and the immunological activity was from 3.10–7.55 IU/mg. The sialic acid content was found to be 1.8–3.2%. Treatment with neuraminidase resulted in a shift of all bands to the alkaline region, however the 7 LH forms were still present.

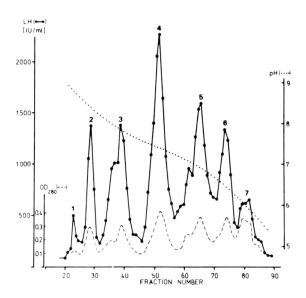

Weise, H. C., D. Graesslin, V. Lichtenberg, G. Rinne: Polymorphism of human pituitary lutropin (LH). (with kind permission of Elsevier Science-NL) FEBS Letters 159 (1983) 93–96.

Fig.2. Preparative isoelectric focusing in sucrose density gradient (440 ml column; pH 4–9.5) of 110 mg purified human pituitary LH complex. Profiles of RIA (——) and UV absorption (– – –) of the different LH isohormones are shown.

48. The complete polymorphism of human pituitary FSH and comparison of the isohormone pattern between males and females

M. Sterneck, D. Graesslin, V. Lichtenberg, G. Bettendorf. *Abt. klinische und experimentelle Endokrinologie, Universitäts-Frauenklinik Hamburg*

Human pituitary follitropin (FSH) has been recognized to be heterogeneous for many years. However, characterization of the hormone polymorphism was incomplete with respect to the number of isohormones as well as to possible qualitative differences between males and females. It was the purpose of this study to demonstrate the complete FSH isohormone system in human pituitaries and, in addition, to compare the FSH forms from males to those of postmenopausal women. Finally, we attempted to obtain further information about the type of microheterogeneity.

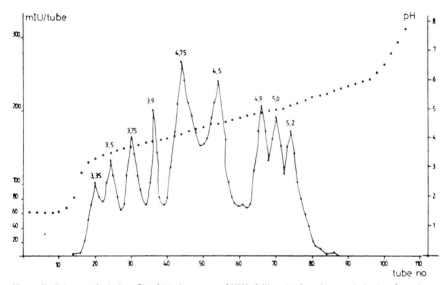

Figure. Radioimmunological profile of 9 isohormones of FSH (follitropin) from human pituitaries after column isoelectric focusing in the pH range 3-6

Sternecke, M., D. Graesslin, V. Lichtenberg, G. Bettendorf: The complete polymorphism of human pituitary FSH and comparison of the isohormone pattern between males and females. Acta endocrinologica 114 (1987) 41–42. (© European J. Endocrinol. formerly Acta endocrinol.).

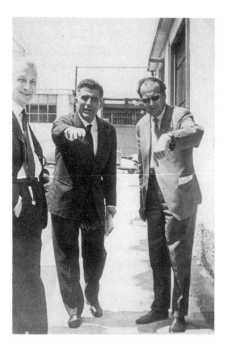

Donini, P.: Entwickelte das erste hMG-Präparat zur klinischen Anwendung in der Firma Serono in Rom, Strukturaufklärung der Gonadotropine. Zusammen mit dem Autor bei der Besichtigung der riesigen Urin-Tanks zur Gonadotropinextraktion (1910).

thus seems appopriate to close this lecture with a reminder of what Shakespeare pointed out in The Tempest „What is past is prologue."

Die ersten Untersuchungen der Gonadotropine mit der Isoelektrofokusierung wurden 1968 auf dem workshop „Gonadotropins 1968" in Vista Hermosa berichtet (*Bettendorf* et al.; *Saxena* und *Rathnam*). *Graesslin* und Mitarbeiter gelang die Aufklärung des Polymorphismus von hCG (*Graesslin* et al., 1972). Mit Hilfe der Gel isoelektrischen Fokussierung konnten fünf hCG-Komponenten isoliert werden. Der Sialinsäuregehalt war unterschiedlich. *Weise* et al. (1983) konnten sieben LH-Isohormone mit der gleichen Methode gewinnen und charakterisieren. Die biologische Wirkung dieser Isohormone wurde durch *Lichtenberg* et al. (1984) untersucht. Aufgrund der Rezeptorbindung, cAMP-Akkumulation und Testosteronproduktion ergab sich „similar intrinsic in vitro biological activity for all isohormones. Quantitatively, however, the potencies of the 7 hormone forms did not correlate with the activities obtained by RIA: there was a dramatic decrease of receptor binding activity compared to immunoactivity from the more alkaline to the more acidic LH isohormones." FSH-Isohormone wurden in der gleichen Arbeitsgruppe untersucht (*Sterneck* et al., 1987). In Hypophysenextrakten konnten neun FSH-Isoformen nachgewiesen werden. Im Gegensatz

Dott. P. DONINI • Dott.ssa R. MONTEZEMOLO

GONADOTROPINA PREIPOFISARIA
E GONADOTROPINA PREIPOFISO-SIMILE UMANA

Estratto dalla " Rassegna di Clinica Terapia e Scienze Affini ,,

Anno XLVIII - Fascicolo IV - Ottobre-Novembre-Dicembre 1949

RÉSUMÉ

Après avoir résumé les principaux caractères biologiques de la gonadotropine pré-hypophysaire, les AA. décrivent les propriétés d'une gonadotropine
qu'ils ont extraite des urines de la ménopause.

En se basant sur les contrôles les plus rigoureux exécutés sur l'action que
cette gonadotropine exerce sur l'appareil sexuel des animaux impubères, les AA.
se croient autorisés à classifier cette gonadotropine comme « gonadotropine pré-
hypophyso-similis humaine » et ils proposent une unité biologique pour son ti-
trage.

On examine ensuite les indications thérapeuthiques de cette hormone.

ISTITUTO NAZIONALE MEDICO FARMACOLOGICO SERONO
ROMA

Donini, P., R. Montezemolo: Gonadotropina preipofisaria e gonadotropina preipofiso-simile
umana. Rassegna die Clinica, Terapia e Science Affini 4 (1949) 1–23.

zum hCG kann der Polymorphismus nicht allein auf den unterschiedlichen Sialinsäuregehalt zurückgeführt werden.

Anreicherungsversuche mit DEAE-Sephadex führten zu höheren biologischen Aktivitäten (*Bettendorf* et al., 1962, *Donini* et al., 1964). Eine weitgehende Trennung von FSH von LH wurde von *Donini* durch immunologische Bindung von LH an Anti-hCG und anschließende DEAE-Cellulose-Chromatographie erreicht. Das erhaltene FSH-Präparat bewirkte keinen Uterusgewichtsanstieg (*Donini* et al., 1966).

Gonadotropinpräparate aus Hypophysen zahlreicher Spezies ergaben spezifische Unterschiede (*Reichert*, 1962, *Walborg* und *Ward*, 1963, *Reichert* und *Parlow*, 1963, *Reichert* und *Jiang*, 1965, *Jutisz* et al., 1965, *Papkoff* et al., 1967). *Reichert* und *Jiang* (1964) verglichen Präparationen von Mensch, Rind, Schwein und Pferd; *Parlow* und *Reichert* (1963) Rind, Schwein, Schaf; *Ward* et al. (1967) Schwein, Rind, Mensch, Ratte und Pferd und *Hartree* et al. von Pferd und Mensch (1968). Die Aminosäure-Zusammensetzung von FSH und von LH aus Hypophysen von Mensch, Schaf, Huhn, Truthahn, Alligator, Schildkröte und Ochsenfrosch weisen eine große Übereinstimmung auf (*Licht*, 1976).

Umfangreiche Studien zur Extraktion und Charakterisierung von Gonadotropinen aus dem Urin wurden vor allem an der Mayo Clinic durchgeführt. Eine ausführliche Diskussion erfolgte auf der Workshop-Conference on Human Pituitary Gonadotropins im Dezember 1959 in Gatlinburg / Tennessee (*Albert*, 1961). Aufgrund der geringen Konzentration im Urin ist eine Anreicherung notwendig. Hierzu wurde herangezogen: Eine Präzipitation mit organischen Lösungsmitteln, wie Ethanol und Aceton; eine Adsorption an Kaolin, Benzoesäure, Aluminiumhydroxid oder Permutit; eine Ultrafiltration (*Albert*, 1955, 1966, *Alexandridis* et al., 1958, *Heinrichs* und *Eulefeld*, 1960, *Keller*, 1963).

Die Extraktion von Gonadotropinen aus Menopausenurin erfolgte mit dem Ziel, ein Präparat für den Einsatz in der Klinik zu gewinnen. *Pietro Donini* schreibt: „Almost immediately after the end of the second World War, in 1947, I entered the field of gonadotropic hormones and I worked on the purification of hCG from human pregnancy urine. I remember that in the library of Serono Institute I read a paper by *Katzman* and *Doisy* on the use of permutit for the purification of hCG; immediately I checked this method and obtained excellent results similar to the authors. … In September 1947 I immediately tried chromatography of menopausal urine through a permutit column. The first experiments were unsuccessful for technical reasons and therefore I changed my strategy and tried to absorb the hormones from menopausal urine with benzoic acid. This method also gave very poor results and therefore I changed the experimental conditions to kaolin as absorbing material instead of the benzoic acid used" (*Donini*, 1995). Die Ergebnisse der ersten Reinigungsversuche wurden 1949 publiziert (*Donini* et al., 1949). Das erste hMG-Präparat „Pergonal" wurde 1950 in Italien eingeführt. Recombinantes humanes FSH mit hoher spezifischer Aktivität und ohne LH-Aktivität wurde durch Einschleusen von humanen FSH-Subunit-Genen in Hamster-Ovarzellen hergestellt (*Keene* et al., 1989, *van Wezenbeek* et al., 1990, *Chappel* et al., 1992). Die ersten klinischen Untersuchungen liegen vor.

Gonadotropin-Therapie

Von historischem Interesse ist der älteste Hinweis auf eine „induzierte Ovulation". *Haighton* beobachtete bei Kaninchen, deren Tuben ligiert waren, nach dem Koitus Ovulationen. „Ovaries can be affected by the stimulus of impregnation without the contact either of palpable semen, or of the aura seminalis" (*Haighton*, 1797). Eine exogene, therapeutische Stimulation der Ovarialfunktion wurde erst durch den Einsatz von Gonadotropinen möglich. Bereits 1934 findet man in einer Übersichtsarbeit aus der Münchener Frauenklinik von *F. G. Dietel* über „Das gonadotrope Hormon des Hypophysen-Vorderlappens" Berichte über die Therapie mit gonadotropen Präparaten. „Zusammenfassend ist zu sagen, daß bei Zyklusstörungen aller Art wohl Erfolge mit Prolan erzielt wurden, daß aber offenbar die Resultate hinter den Erwartungen zurückstehen, welche man in Kenntnis der biologischen Wirkungen des gon. H. beim Tier hegen möge." In dem 385 Titel umfassenden Literaturverzeichnis betreffen 35 die Therapie (*Dietel*, 1934).

Bevor Präparate mit gonadotroper Aktivität zur Verfügung standen, wurden tierische Hypophysen transplantiert. *Eskil Kylin* (1935) an der inneren Abteilung des allgemeinen Krankenhaus zu Jönköping in Schweden, meinte bei der Simmond'schen Kachexie einen Effekt gesehen zu haben. 24 Patienten wurden „Kalbshypophysen implantiert, die in mehrere kleine Teile zerschnitten waren, um auf diese Weise ein Festwachsen besser zu gewährleisten. ... Ein 19jähriger Mann, der an Dystrophia adiposogenitalis litt, war 5 Monate nach der Operation vollständig genesen. Die Testes waren von Erbsen- bis zu Taubeneiergröße gewachsen. ... Bei 23 Kranken handelte es sich um Simmondsche Krankheit. 12 Kranke sind vollkommen geheilt." Dagegen *A. Westman* „Die Erfolge waren schlecht. Klar ist bei dieser Methode von vornherein, daß man nur eine vorübergehende hormonale Beeinflussung des Krankheitsgeschehens erreichen wird. Selbst dann, wenn es zur Einheilung des Implantats kommt, so kann immer nur die zur Zeit der Implantation in der Hypophyse gespeicherte und dann resorbierte Hormonmenge wirksam werden." *Westman* untersuchte ein Implantat und fand nur nekrotisches, ab-

Ergebnisse.

(Aus der Univ.-Frauenklinik, München. — Direktor: Prof. Dr. H. Eymer.)

Das gonadotrope Hormon des Hypophysen-Vorderlappens.

Von

Privatdozent Dr. **F. G. Dietel.**

Die Versuche, durch Zufuhr von Vorderlappen- (VL.-) Substanz den Zustand der Keimdrüsen und den Cyclus bei Nagern zu beeinflussen, gehen bis ins Jahr 1916 zurück (Goetsch[1], Long und Evans[2]). Einen großen Aufschwung hat die Erforschung der VL.-Substanzen jedoch erst in den letzten Jahren erfahren infolge der Entdeckung des gonadotropen Hormons (gon. H.) durch Aschheim[3] und Zondek[4]*, Smith[5] sowie Long und Evans[6]. Die hierüber fast aus allen Ländern der Erde erschienene Literatur ist ins Ungeheuere gewachsen. Da Zondek und Aschheim das gon. H. auch in der Placenta und vor allem im Schwangerenurin nachweisen konnten, das Problem, ob die wirksamen Stoffe in VL., Placenta und Urin identisch seien, jedoch heute noch nicht gelöst ist, scheint es erforderlich, auch das im Mutterkuchen vorhandene sowie das im Harn ausgeschiedene Hormon (Prolan) in diese Betrachtungen einzubeziehen.

I. Wirkung des gon. H. auf das Nagerovar.

Bei den im Laboratorium benutzten Nagern ruft das gon.H. im Kurzversuch bekanntlich 3 Wirkungen am Ovarium, besonders auch jenem infantiler (inf.) Tiere, hervor:

Die Hypophysenvorderlappenreaktion I (HVR. I) = Follikelreifung durch HVH. A.

Die Hypophysenvorderlappenreaktion II (HVR. II) = Bildung von Blutpunkten.

Die Hypophysenvorderlappenreaktion III (HVR. III) = Corpora lutea durch HVH. B.

Die HVR. II wird nach Aschheim durch gleichzeitige Wirkung von HVH. A und B ausgelöst, jedoch hält es Zondek für möglich, daß sie durch HVH. A allein entstehen kann. Das Vorhandensein reifer Follikel führt bei Nagern sekundär zum prämenstruellen Aufbau der Uterusschleimhaut und Oestrus (Schollenstadium), Erscheinungen, die auch durch Follikulinzufuhr ausgelöst werden können. Während letzteres aber auch am kastrierten Tier seine Wirkung entfaltet, beeinflußt das gon. H. nur den Uterus und die Scheide intakter Tiere auf dem Umweg über das Ovar. Nach Dauerzufuhr von gon. H. stellen sich bei intakten inf. und auch geschlechtsreifen Tieren verschiedene Reaktionen ein, die vom Gehalt der injizierten Lösungen an HVH. A und B abhängig sind; sie verschwinden nach 3—4 Wochen wieder (Zondek[7]). Die unter dem Einfluß von HVH. A aus den prämaturen Follikeln des inf. Nagerovars ausgestoßenen Eier sind nicht befruchtungsfähig (Aschheim und Zondek, Ehrhardt[8], Siegmund[95]). Man erzielt also keine wirkliche Frühreife, es fehlt die aus unbekannten Einflüssen herrührende somatische Reife (Engle[9]). Dagegen müssen die experimentell hervorgerufenen Corpora lutea (atretica) als funktionstüchtig angesprochen werden aus folgenden Gründen: 1. Um einen in den Uterus des Versuchstieres eingebrachten Seidenfaden bilden sich Deciduazellwucherungen (Placentome [Evans

---

* Die Arbeiten von Aschheim und Zondek werden nur einzeln aufgeführt, soweit die darin enthaltenen Ergebnisse nicht in [3] oder [4] niedergelegt sind.

Dietel, F. G.: Das gonadotrope Hormon des Hypophysen-Vorderlappens. Berichte über die gesamte Gynäkologie und Geburtshilfe sowie deren Grenzgebiete 27 (1934) 369–448.

ERGEBNISSE VON 24 HYPOPHYSEN-TRANSPLANTATIONEN.

Von

ESKIL KYLIN.

Aus der Inneren Abteilung des allgemeinen Krankenhauses zu Jönköping (Schweden).

Nr.	Alter	Anamnese	Befund	R. R.	Blutzucker in mg %	Grundumsatz	Körpergewicht in kg	Körperlänge	Nachuntersuchungen Befund	R. R.	Blutzucker in mg %	Grundumsatz	Körpergewicht in kg	Zunahme des Körpergewichtes	Observation in Monaten
1	18	Krank seit 2 Jahren. Appetitlosigkeit. Müdigkeit. Schwindel. Obstipation. Kopfschmerz. Abmagerung. Frostgefühl.	Hochgradig abgemagert. Subnormale Temperatur. Pigmentierungen. Operiert Nov. 1934. Psychisch abnorm.	70	75 (42)	−40	33	162	Wurde vollständig gesund und arbeitsfähig als Landarbeiterin. Menstruiert normal seit April 1936. Psychisch vollständig normal.	125	—	−8	63	30	20
2	47	Seit 5 Jahren immer kränker. Müdigkeit. Appetitlosigkeit. Kopfschmerz. Schwindel. Hypoglykämisches Koma. Schlaflosigkeit. Nervös. Amenorrhöe. Obstipation. Frostgefühl.	Braungelbliche Pigmentierung. Mager. Operiert Dez. 1934.	80	42	−18	56	—	Wurde klinisch gesund. Starb 7 Monate nach der Operation an Pneumonie. Hypophyse atrophisch, bindegewebig induriert. Basophile Zellen sehr spärlich. Eosinophile Zellen und Hauptzellen zahlreich.	110	104	+16	—	—	7
3	50	Krank seit 10 Jahren. Müdigkeit. Schlaflosigkeit. Abmagerung. Kopfschmerz. Obstipation. Frostgefühl.	Pigmentiert. Sehr mager. Kachektisch. Operiert Febr. 1935.	80	78	−35	43	—	Wurde klinisch gesund und arbeitsfähig. Starb an Pneumonie 14 Monate nach der Operation. Die Hypophyse war mehr als doppelt groß. Keine reifen basophilen Zellen. Reichlich eosinophile Zellen. Der Tumor bestand zum größten Teil aus Hauptzellen.	—	—	−2	46	3	13
4	42	Krank seit 5 Jahren. Adynamie. Schwindel. Abmagerung. Dysmenorrhöe.	Operiert April 1935.	100	95	−13	48	—	Wurde vollständig gesund und arbeitsfähig als Lehrerin.	—	—	—	52	4	14
5	25	Krank seit 4—5 Jahren. Schlaflosigkeit. Abmagerung. Adynamie. Appetitlosigkeit. Amenorrhöe. Schwindel. Kopfschmerzen. Frostgefühl.	Pigmentiert. Sehr mager. Operiert Mai 1935.	60	82	−43	41,3	164	Wurde vollständig gesund und arbeitsfähig als Lehrerin. Psychisch vollständig normal. Menstruiert normal seit Dez. 1935.	120	99	−16	58,5	17,2	13
6	23	Wog mit 17 Jahren 60 kg. Versuchte abzumagern. Dann magerte sie stark ab, wurde appetitlos, müde und elend. Amenorrhöe. Kopfschmerz. Schwindel. Frostgefühl.	Abgemagert. Kachektisch. Pigmentiert. Psychisch sehr schwer zu behandeln. Suicidversuch. Operiert Juli 1935.	70	68	−44	30,5	166	Wurde deutlich gebessert.	100	82	−23	37	6,5	12
7	22	Krank seit 2 Jahren. Wog damals 70 kg. Müdigkeit. Abmagerung. Appetitlosigkeit. Schwindel. Kopfschmerz. Amenorrhöe. Suicidversuch.	Pigmentiert. Abgemagert. Elend. Psychisch sehr auffällig. Körpertemperatur um 36—36,5°. Operiert Aug. 1935.	85	50	−53	40,8	172	Wurde vollständig gesund und arbeitsfähig. Psychisch vollständig normal.	90	110	−18	55	14,2	11
8	22	Krank seit 6 Jahren. Wog damals 50 kg. Appetitlosigkeit. Abmagerung. Adynamie. Frösteln.	Pigmentiert. Sehr mager. Kachektisch. Operiert Aug. 1935.	90	85	−9	40	164	Zuerst gebessert und arbeitsfähig. 5—6 Monate nach der Operation wieder krank mit Diarrhöe und Magenbeschwerden. Klinisch Gärungsdyspepsie.	120	85	+4	46	6	11
9	30	Seit 3 Jahren krank. Früheres Körpergewicht 62 kg. Appetitlosigkeit. Abmagerung. Adynamie. Kopfschmerz. Schwindel. Magenbeschwerden. Schlaflosigkeit. Amenorrhöe. Seit einem Jahr zu Bett. Psychisch auffällig.	Pigmentiert. Abgemagert. Kachektisch. Subnormale Temp. Operiert Aug. 1935.	90	62	−50	25,5	160	Wurde gebessert. Beschäftigt mit kleinen Handarbeiten. Macht kleine Spaziergänge. Appetit recht gut. Psychisch gebessert, aber noch „nervös".	—	—	—	38,5	13	11
10	19	Krank seit 2 Jahren. Früheres Körpergewicht 60 kg. Appetitlosigkeit. Abmagerung. Adynamie. Frösteln. Amenorrhöe. Magenbeschwerden. Kopfschmerz. Deprimiert.	Pigmentiert. Kachektisch. Abgemagert. Subnormale Temp. Operiert Okt. 1935.	60	64	−44	31,5	169	Wurde vollständig gesund und arbeitsfähig (Studentin).	125	100	−18	48	16,5	9

Zusammenfassung: Bericht über 24 Kranke, die mit Transplantation von Kalbshypophyse behandelt wurden.

Ein 19jähr. Mann, der an Dystrophia adiposogenitalis litt, war 5 Monate nach der Operation vollständig gesu..d geworden. Die Testes waren von Erbsen- bis zu Taubeneier- größe gewachsen. Die Fettansammlung von weiblichem Typus war verschwunden, und der Patient sah männlich aus, Bart- und Pubeshaare waren gewachsen.

Bei 23 Kranken handelte es sich um Simmondssche Krankheit. 12 Kranke sind vollkommen geheilt. Das Körpergewicht stieg an, bei einem Falle um 30 kg. Bei 6 Fällen war eine deutliche Besserung festzustellen. Da bei diesen Kranken die Zeit zu kurz ist, können die endgültigen Ergebnisse noch nicht beurteilt werden. 2 Kranke sind ge- storben, ohne daß eine Besserung eintrat, und zwar ein Kranker unmittelbar und ein anderer 3 Monate nach der Operation. 3 Kranke sind so frisch operiert, daß eine Bewertung des Erfolges nicht möglich ist.

Kylin, E.: Ergebnis- se von 24 Hypophy- sen-Transplantatio- nen (© Springer- Verlag). Klin. Wo- chenschr. 15 (1936) 1757–1760.

gekapseltes, nicht vaskularisiertes Gewebe. *A. Vöge* in Heidelberg implantier- te frische Kalbshypophysen. „Die Erfolge waren schlecht" (1943).

Campbell und *Collip* berichteten 1930 über die orale Verabreichung von Plazentaextrakten an drei Patienten. Bei zwei Amenorrhoen kam es zu Blu- tungen, eine Dysmenorrhö verschwand.

Um 1930 wurden die ersten therapeutischen Versuche mit Urinextrak- ten und mit Schwangerenblut durchgeführt. Zunächst versuchte man die ju- venile Dauerblutung zu behandeln. „With strongly luteinizing preparations, it has been possible to check functional hemorrhage in 27 of 29 cases. In 14 of our 51 cases the bleeding has ceased after a single injection, and in 12 af- ter two injections" (*Novak* und *Hurd*, 1931). Durch die Verabreichung go- nadotroper Aktivität im Schwangerenblut hoffte man, den persistierenden Follikel zur Ovulation zu bringen. Mit der Bluttransfusion konnte gleichzei- tig die bestehende Anämie beeinflußt werden. „Wenn meine Voraussetzun- gen richtig sind, so muß der durch Schwangerenbluttransfusion einen akuten Hormonstoß erhaltende pathologische Follikel im Ovarium zum mindesten gestört, wahrscheinlich luteinisiert werden. Dann müßte sich infolgedessen im Uterus die Schleimhaut in eine Sekretionsphase verwandeln und nach Ablaufen der Corpus luteum-Wirkung die Schleimhaut im Menstruations- prozeß abgehen. Dazu kann ich sagen, daß mehrfach auf die fast momentan eintretende Blutstillung und auf ein anschließendes 6–10 Tage währendes völlig blutfreies Intervall eine schwache, menstruationsähnliche Blutung ein- setzte und dementsprechend von selbst nach einigen Tagen wieder ver- schwand" (*Clauberg*, 1933). Die Ergebnisse der Verabreichung von Prolan

A, d.h. dem Chorionhormon ergaben, daß dies sich „durch einige Eigenschaften von dem gonadotropen Hormon, das die Hypophyse abgibt, unterscheidet" (*Westman*, 1937). „Mit Prolan A scheint man keine Follikelreifung, aber in gewissen Fällen Luteinisierungsprozesse auslösen zu können." *Büttner* konnte bei 17 von 23 persistenten Follikeln eine Luteinisierung beobachten. Ihn interessierte die Frage, ob durch die Gonadotropinpräparate möglicherweise eine Schädigung der Ovarien eintreten könne. „Eine Schädigung der Ovarien im Sinne einer vermehrten Follikelatresie oder der Unterdrückung zyklischer Vorgänge wurde in keinem Fall beobachtet" (*Büttner*, Habilitationsschrift, Bonn, 1937). *Zondek* faßte 1936 zusammen: „Die bisherige Hormontherapie war eine hormonale Ersatztherapie an der Verbrauchsstätte, das Ziel der Hormontherapie muß die hormonotrope Stimulationstherapie an der Produktionsstätte sein. ... Das Prolan wirkt, wie aus den mitgeteilten Beobachtungen hervorgeht, auch beim Menschen gonadotrop, es vermag das noch nicht funktionierende Ovarium anzukurbeln, das funktionierende Ovarium zu erhöhter Funktion anzuregen und das nicht mehr funktionierende zu reaktivieren" (*Zondek*, 1936).

Browne und *Venning* berichteten 1938 über eine gesteigerte und verlängerte Pregnandiol-Ausscheidung und eine Verschiebung der nachfolgenden Menstruation, wenn hCG in der Lutealphase eines normalen Zyklus verabreicht wurde. Die physiologische Wirkung auf das Corpus luteum von Affen wurde von *Hisaw* (1944) untersucht und eine Verlängerung der Lutealphase beobachtet.

Die Wirkung von hCG bei normalen Frauen wurde von *Brown* und *Bradbury* untersucht (1947). „hCG ist luteotrophic in women and will induce a pseudopregnant condition, as evidenced by a prolongation of the functional life of the corpus luteum, the development of a decidua, and the prolonged excretion of pregnanediol. .. Until objective evidence of other gonadotrophic action in women is obtained, the use of hCG should be directed toward the maintenance or augmentation of luteal function."

Eine umfangreiche Studie über die Behandlung der Metropathia haemoragica cystica mit hCG erschien 1950 von *T. Wahlén*: „During the 10 year period 1939–1948 there were 563 cases of metropathia haemoragica cystica treated at the Women's Clinic in Malmö. In this work these have been brought together and analysed with reference to symptomatology, course, prognosis, and treatment – especially hormonal therapy with chorionic gonadotrophin" (*Wahlen*, 1950). Neben der Beschreibung von Blutungen in den verschiedenen Lebensphasen, wird über 28 Fälle berichtet, bei denen die Blutung im Zusammenhang mit einer Östrogenmedikation auftrat. Die Indi-

A STUDY OF THE PHYSIOLOGIC ACTION OF HUMAN CHORIONIC HORMONE*

The Production of Pseudopregnancy in Women by Chorionic Hormone

W. E. BROWN, M.D., AND J. T. BRADBURY, SC.D., IOWA CITY, IOWA

(From the Department of Obstetrics and Gynecology, State University of Iowa)

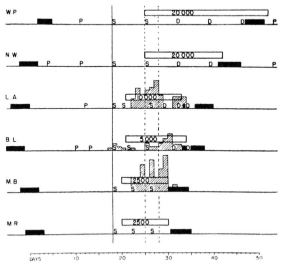

Fig. 1.—Graphic representation of the observations on six subjects in whom treatment was started in the premenstrual (luteal) phase of the cycle. The black bars represent menstruation. The letters represent endometrial biopsies, *P* for proliferative, *S* for secretory, *D* for decidual reaction, and *R* for resting. The vertical line indicates the date of the first secretory biopsy, and the vertical broken lines the approximate interval of expected menstruation. The open bars indicate the duration of treatment, and the numbers denote the dosage of chorionic hormone in I.U. per day. The shaded bars represent the excretion of pregnanediol in mg. per day.

Brown, W. E., J. T. Bradbury: A study of the physiologic action of human chorionic hormone. (permission granted by Mosby-Year Book, Inc. St. Louis, MO, USA) Am. J. Obst. & Gynec. 53 (1947) 749–757.

kation für die Östrogensubstitution waren klimakterische Beschwerden, Polyarthritis, klimakterische Arthritis sowie eine Augenerkrankung und Endometritis.

Die Therapie der funktionellen Blutungen bestand in Röntgen-Kastration, Curettage, zyklischer Östrogen-Gestagen- oder hCG-(Pregnyl-)Verabreichung. Pregnyl wurde in insgesamt 53 Fällen verabreicht. „It was not employed for haemostatic purposes, the objective being instead to restore ovulatory cycles and to preclude recurrence. ... 38 (= 82.6%) responded to the therapy by showing diphasic basal temperature, secretory change of the endometrium and normal menstruations. ... The material in its entirety shows that chorionic gonadotrophin can be used – with very great prospects of a good result (probable or certain ovulatory cycles) – as a substitution or stimulation therapy (as regards of the ovaries) for even severe m. h. c. cases in the fertile age with a considerable tendency to recurrence" (*Wahlén*, 1950).

A. Palmer (1957) behandelte 84 sterile Frauen mit einer Corpus luteum-Insuffizienz mit hCG Injektionen post-ovulatorisch. Bei 53 Patienten trat eine Schwangerschaft entweder im Therapiezyklus oder im Folgezyklus ein. „hCG in the dosage used (1000 i. u.) was 100 % effective in prolonging the „highphase" of the basal body temperature and in delaying the onset of the menses for at least 14 days."

In einem Vortrag der deutsch-schweizerischen Gynäkologischen Gesellschaft im November 1960 in Bern berichtete *P. Muller* über „Vor- und Nachteile der hochkonzentrierten Choriongonadotropin-Präparate". Die von *M. F. Jayle* bezeichnete dynamische Untersuchung des Corpus luteum betrifft die Verabreichung von zwei Ampullen zu 10 000 IE eines Choriongonadotropin-Präparates in einem Abstand von 48 Stunden. Eine Dosierung der Harnsteroide erfolgt sieben Tage später und ergibt wertvolle Schlußfolgerungen über die Gelbkörperfunktion. Dieses Verfahren ist einfach und gefahrlos. Hingegen kann die therapeutische Gabe von hochkonzentrierten serischen und Choriongonadotropin-Präparaten zur Behandlung einer Amenorrhö, falls eine polizystische Dystrophie der Ovarien besteht, zu dramatischen Ovarialrupturen führen (*Muller* 1961).

Uneinheitliche Reaktionen erzielte man mit der intramuskulären und auch intravenösen Verabreichung von Urinextrakten.

Extrakte aus tierischen Hypophysen wurden noch bis Anfang der 60er Jahre zur Therapie eingesetzt. *Georgeanna Seegar Jones* behandelte 40 amenorrhoische Patienten mit einem Extrakt aus Pferde-Hypophysen (*Squibb* und *Sons,* New York). Zwei Schwangerschaften resultierten, 21 Ovulationen, drei Blutungen und 14 ohne Reaktion (*Jones* et al., 1961). In der Zusammenfassung dieser Arbeit schreiben die Autoren: „The human ovary is responsive to sheep pituitary gonadotrophin ..." und „there is some clinical evidence in this series that refractoriness to gonadotrophins of animal origin develops after repeated administration even though the duration of the initial administration may be very short."

Dörner und *Daume* (1961) setzten „Folistiman", ein von *Schäfer* (1961) im Arzneimittelwerk Dresden hergestelltes Präparat mit follikelstimulierender Wirkung aus Schweinehypophysen, ein und konnten Ovarialstimulationen erzielen. *Groot-Wassink* verglich die Wirkung dieses tierischen Präparates mit humanem FSH (1967) und fand, daß ersteres zu besseren Resultaten, gemessen an der Schwangerschaftsrate, führte. Als Ursache wurde das verschiedene FSH/LH-Verhältnis der beiden Extrakte angenommen. Das humane FSH hatte die Relation FSH/LH von 11:1 und das tierische von 70:1.

Cole und *Hart* hatten 1930 gonadotrope Aktivität im Serum schwangerer Stuten nachgewiesen. 1943 konnten *Cole* und *Goss* zeigen, daß als Bildungsort besondere Strukturen des Endometriums gelten, die sog. „endometrial cups". Das Stutenserumgonadotropin oder pregnant mare serum gonadotrophin (PMSG) wurde von *Engle* und *Hamburger* an juvenilen Affen getestet. Der Effekt war eine Follikelreifung ohne Corpus luteum-Bildung vergleichbar der Wirkung von Extrakten aus dem Urin von kastrierten Frauen, deren „Identität mit dem Vorderlappenhormon" bekannt war. *A. Westman* untersuchte die Wirkung von „Antex", einem PMSG-Präparat der *A. G. Leo*, Hälsingborg, bei „Frauen mit normaler Menstruation", „die wegen Geistesschwäche sterilisiert werden sollten" und bei Myomen. „Die Wirkung des Antex auf die Ovarien der Frau gleicht der, die man bei Affenovarien gefunden hat, außerordentlich stark" (*Westman*, 1937). *M. Edward Davis* und *Arthur K. Koff* im Chicago Lying in Hospital berichteten auf dem Annual Meeting der Central Association of Obstetricians and Gynecologists im Oktober 1937 in Dallas/Texas: „It has been possible for the first time to produce ovulation in women by the intravenous use of gonadotropic hormone derived from serum of pregnant mares. This hormone has been isolated in such an advanced state of purity that its administration by the i.m. or i.v. route is devoid of danger, provided that suitable safegards are established. Biological, this gonadotropic hormone resembles extracts and implants of the anterior lobe of the hypophysis but differs chemically and biologically from all other gonadotropic substances heretofore studied." *Rydberg* und Østergaard (1939) beschrieben die Wirkung einer Antex-Physex-Behandlung bei amenorrhoischen Frauen. Von 27 sekundären Amenorrhoen reagierten 22 mit einer Menstruationsblutung, von sechs primären Amenorrhoen drei. In der Arbeit „Effect of Serum Gonadotropin und Chorionic Gonadotropin on the Human Ovary" von *Rydberg* und *Pedersen-Bjergaard* (1943) ist die Östrogenausscheidung während der Behandlung untersucht worden. Zwei Fälle mit Ovarialvergrößerung werden berichtet: „The treatment may give some untoward effects, the most important of which is the not altogether infrequent production of a considerable swelling of one of the ovaries or of both. ... In one case we were able during a laparotomy to ascertain that it was a matter of lutein tumors." Die Autoren erwähnen in der Einleitung, „in June 1940 the Council of Pharmacy and Chemistry of the American Medical Association published a report in which is said in conclu-

American Journal of
Obstetrics and Gynecology

| VOL. 36 | AUGUST, 1938 | No. 2 |

Central Association of Obstetricians and Gynecologists
Ninth Annual Meeting, October 14 to 16, 1937
Dr. Jean P. Pratt, of Detroit, Presiding

THE EXPERIMENTAL PRODUCTION OF OVULATION IN THE HUMAN SUBJECT*†

M. EDWARD DAVIS, M.D., AND ARTHUR K. KOFF, M.D., CHICAGO, ILL.

(From the Department of Obstetrics and Gynecology, The University of Chicago and The Chicago Lying-in Hospital)

CONCLUSIONS

1. It has been possible for the first time to produce ovulation in women by the intravenous use of a gonadotropic hormone derived from serum of pregnant mares.

2. This hormone has been isolated in such an advanced state of purity that its administration by the intramuscular or intravenous route is devoid of danger, provided that suitable safeguards are established.

3. Biologically, this gonadotropic hormone resembles extracts and implants of the anterior lobe of the hypophysis but differs chemically and biologically from all other gonadotropic substances heretofore studied.

4. These experimental ovulations have provided the earliest human corpora lutea yet described.

5. Clinically, this gonadotropic hormone should prove efficacious in the therapy of patients in whom follicle growth and ovulation are at fault.

Literaturverzeichnis*. (385 Titel !!)
Teil I.

[1] Goetsch, Bull. Hopkins Hosp. 27, 29 (1916). — [2] Long u. Evans, Proc. nat. Acad. Sci. U.S.A. 8, 38 (1922). — [3] Aschheim, Die Schwangerschaftsdiagnose aus dem Harn. Berlin 1933. — [4] Zondek, B., Die Hormone des Ovariums und des Hypophysenvorderlappens. Berlin 1931. — [5] Smith, Proc. Soc. exper. Biol. a. Med. 24, 131 (1926); 561 (1927) — Amer. J. Physiol. 80, 114 (1927). — [6] Long u. Evans, Anat. Rec. 21, 62 (1921); 23, 19 (1922). — [7] Zondek, Klin. Wschr. 1933 I, 857. — [8] Ehrhardt, Arch. Gynäk. 148, 235 (1932). — [9] Engle, Endocrinology 15, 405 (1931). — [10] Evans u. Simpson, Proc. Soc.

---

* Es konnte nur die bis Ende 1933 erschienene Literatur berücksichtigt werden.

Davis, M. E., A. Koff: The experimental production of ovulation in the human subject. (permission granted Mosby Year Book) Am. J. Obst. Gynec. 36 (1938) 183–199

(FROM GYNAECOLOGICAL WARD I, RIGSHOSPITALET, COPENHAGEN: SENIOR
PHYSICIAN: PROFESSOR ERIK RYDBERG, M. D.)

The effect of gonadotropic hormone treatment in cases of amenorrhoea. [1]

Production of true menstruation and increased excretion of oestrin.

By

ERIK RYDBERG and ERLING ØSTERGAARD.

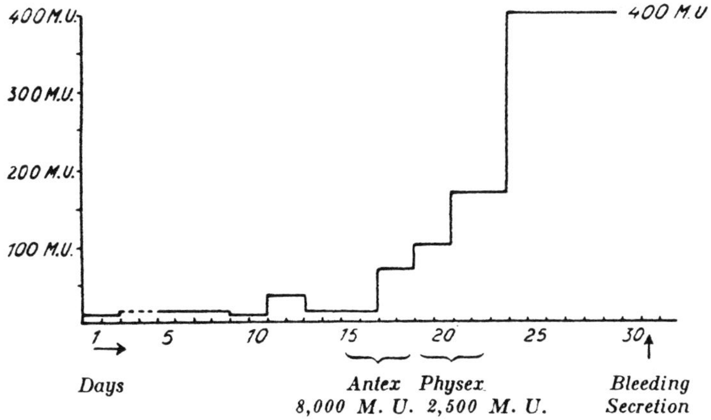

Diagram I. Treatment and excretion of oestrin.

E.C.O. 18 years old. Amenorrhoea 1 ½ years. True menstruation at typical moment after treatment. Regular menstruation since, lasting 4—5 days, at monthly intervals. Under observation for 9 months.

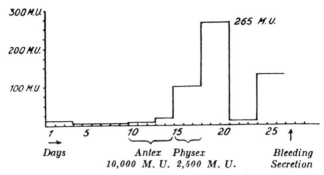

Diagram II. Treatment and excretion of oestrin.
K. M. S. 24 years old. Amenorrhoea 6 years. True menstruation at typical
moment after treatment. This patient did not continue to menstruate spon-
taneously.

Rydberg, E., E. Østergaard: The effect of gonadotropic hormone treatment in cases of amenorrhoea. (© Munksgaard Int. Publisher Ltd. Copenhagen, Denmark) Acta Obstet. Gyn. Scand. 19
(1939) 222–246.

sion that the treatment of ovarian disturbances with chorionic gonadotropin
for the present has no rational foundation" (Report of the Council of Pharmacy and Chemistry of the American Medical Association, 1940).

A. *Vöge* berichtet ausführlich über die intravenöse Verabreichung von
Anteron (Schering) bei zystisch glandulärer Hyperplasie. Da „wir im Stuten-
serum kein absolut ideales Mittel besitzen, um den Follikelsprung auszulö-
sen, weil die A- und B-Komponenten nicht im richtigen Verhältnis zueinan-
der abgestimmt sind, haben ‚wir‘, … daher nach einer Möglichkeit gesucht,
in die bisher beschriebene Form der Therapie eine unterstützende bzw. zusätzliche Behandlung einzubauen und sind bei dieser Überlegung auf das
Corpusluteum gekommen." 10 mg Progesteron in 1 ml wurden intrauterin
gleichzeitig mit Anteron i.v. verabreicht. „Mit dieser Behandlung, zur rech-
ten Zeit begonnen, sind wir in der Lage, jede Metropathieblutung im gün-
stigsten Sinne zu beeinflussen. Es gibt keine Zufallstreffer mehr" (*Vöge,*
1943).

„Die Aussichten auf Erfolg der Hormonbehandlung der als funktionelle
weibliche Sterilität diagnostizierten Fälle wird zur Zeit mit 20–30 Prozent
veranschlagt" (*Rydberg* und *Madsen,* 1949). Von *Hamblen* und *Davis* wurde
1945 die „one-two cyclic gonadotropic therapy" beschrieben: PMS vom 5.
bis 14. Tag, hCG vom 15. bis 24. Tag. „The following conclusions appear
warranted:

AMERICAN JOURNAL OF OBSTETRICS AND GYNECOLOGY

TREATMENT OF HYPOOVARIANISM BY THE SEQUENTIAL AND CYCLIC ADMINISTRATION OF EQUINE AND CHORIONIC GONADOTROPINS—SO-CALLED ONE-TWO CYCLIC GONADOTROPIC THERAPY

Summary of Five Years' Results*

E. C. HAMBLEN, M.D., AND C. D. DAVIS, M.D., DURHAM, N. C.

(From the Endocrine Division of the Department of Obstetrics and Gynecology, Duke University School of Medicine and Duke Hospital)

THE first series of so-called one-two cyclic gonadotropic therapy was administered, during the latter part of October and the first part of November of 1939, to a patient with ovarian sterility, who became pregnant during the treatment. Details of this therapeutic schedule and the history of this patient were reported by one of us (E. C. H.) about the middle of November, 1939, at the annual meeting of the Southern Medical Association in Memphis, Tennessee. At this time, it was stated that the sequential and cyclic employment of equine and chorionic gonadotropins warranted further and more intensive study. Subsequently, our group gave reports upon results of this therapeutic

*This study was aided by grants to one of us (E.C.H.) as follows: From the Research Council of Duke University; from Ayerst, McKenna & Harrison, Ltd., Montreal, Canada; from Schering Corporation, Bloomfield, N. J.; from The Upjohn Company, Kalamazoo, Mich.; and from the National Committee on Maternal Health, New York, N. Y. Preparations of equine gonadotropin included Anteron (Schering Corporation) and Gonadogen (Upjohn Company); those of chorionic gonadotropin included APL (Ayerst, McKenna & Harrison) and chorionic gonadotropin (Upjohn Company).

Hamblen, E. C., C. D. Davis, N. C. Durham: Treatment of hypoovarianism y the sequential and cyclic administration of equine and chorionic gonadotropins – so-called one-two cyclic gonadotropic therapy. (Permission by Mosby-Year Book, Inc., St. Louis, Mo, USA) Am. J. Obstet. Gynecol. 50 (1945) 137–146.

1. Patients with hypooestrogenism respond poorly to this system of gonadotropic therapy.

2. Patients with anovulatory failure without hypooestrogenism respond well to this system of therapy.

3. A small percentage of sterile women, whose bleeding from progestional endometrium constitutes the only significant finding upon their surveys or those of their husbands, become pregnant when treated with one-two cyclic gonadotropic therapy."

O. Riisfeldt berichtete 1949 über eine zwölf Jahresperiode einer Gonadotropinbehandlung bei Amenorrhö und Sterilität. 117 Fälle von Amenorrhö wurden behandelt. „In den meisten Fällen von sekundärer Amenorrhö ist es möglich das ruhende Ovarium wieder zur Funktion zu bringen oder wenig-

Summary and Conclusions

A total of 116 hypoovarian patients, whose ages placed them in the adolescent or reproductive epochs, was treated by the sequential and cyclic administration of equine and chorionic gonadotropins. The following results were obtained:

1. Only one of seven patients with deficient sexual maturation and non-occurrence of menarche (hypoestrogenism) yielded a progestational endometrium during therapy.

2. Four of thirteen patients, or 30.8 per cent, with infrequent and/or scanty estrogenic uterine bleeding yielded progestational endometriums during therapy.

3. Fifteen of thirty-one patients, or 48.5 per cent, with prolonged and/or excessive estrogenic bleeding yielded progestational endometriums during therapy.

4. Seven of fourteen patients, or 50 per cent, with cyclic estrogenic bleeding and ovarian sterility yielded positive responses, including four pregnancies, during therapy.

5. Nine of fifty patients, or 18 per cent, with cyclic bleeding from immature progestational endometriums became pregnant during therapy.

The following conclusions appear warranted:

1. Patients with hypoestrogenism (as illustrated by those with deficient sexual maturation) respond poorly to this system of gonadotropic therapy.

2. Patients with anovulatory ovarian failure without hypoestrogenism (as illustrated by those with diverse types of estrogenic bleeding) respond well to this system of therapy: a total of 44.8 per cent yielded progestational endometriums.

3. A small percentage (18 per cent) of sterile women, whose bleeding from immature progestational endometriums constitutes the only significant finding upon their surveys or those of their husbands, become pregnant when treated with one-two cyclic gonadotropic therapy.

Hamblen, E. C., C. D. Davis, N. C. Durham: Treatment of hypoovarianism y the sequential and cyclic administration of equine and chorionic gonadotropins – so-called one-two cyclic gonadotropic therapy. (Permission by Mosby-Year Book, Inc., St. Louis, Mo, USA) Am. J. Obstet. Gynecol. 50 (1945) 137–146.

Nicht einzeln im Buchhandel käuflich

Sonderdruck aus „Zeitschrift für Geburtshilfe und Gynäkologie"

156. Band, 2. Heft, Seite 144—157. 1961

Herausgegeben von

Prof. Dr. E. P h i l i p p in Kiel und Prof. Dr. H. H u b e r in Marburg/L.

F e r d i n a n d E n k e V e r l a g S t u t t g a r t

Aus der Univ.-Frauenklinik Kiel (Direktor: Prof. Dr. E. P h i l i p p)

Über die Zyklusinduktion exogener Gonadotropine (PMS und HCG)

(Ein klinischer Beitrag zum Synergismus zwischen Hypophysenfunktion und Choriongonadotropin) *)

Von **H.-J. Staemmler**

Mit 8 Abbildungen

Herrn Geheimrat Prof. Dr. med., Dr. med. h. c., Dr. jur. h. c. W a l t e r S t o e c k e l zur Vollendung des 90. Lebensjahres in Verehrung zugeeignet.

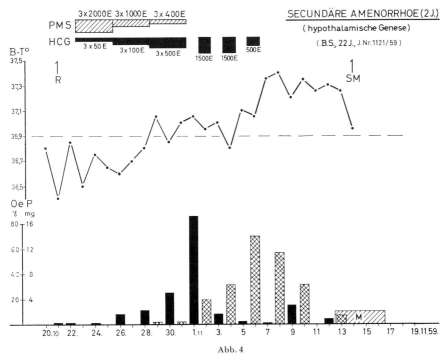

Abb. 4

stens für eine Zeit lang, durch eine kombinierte Behandlung mit Serum- und Choriongonadotropin. ... Die wirksamste Form für Behandlung ist wie folgt: Antex (Serumgonadotropin) 3000 i. E. täglich in fünf aufeinander folgenden Tagen, und danach Physex (Choriongonadotropin) 1500 i. E. jeden zweiten Tag, im ganzen drei Injektionen. Gewöhnlich tritt dann die Menstruation am 8.–10. Tag nach der letzten Injektion ein. ... Primäre Amenorrhö gibt im allgemeinen ganz schlechte Aussichten für Erfolg. ... Es wird erwähnt, daß Gravidität oft nach der Behandlung von Amenorrhö bei sterilen Patienten folgt" (*Riisfeldt*, 1949). *Igarashi* und *Matsumoto* weisen auf die Bedeutung der individualisierten Therapie hin und beschreiben die Zervixsekretion als guten Parameter der Follikelreife (1957). „The essentials of this method lie in (1) the administration of pregnant mare serum so as to make the follicle mature, (2) the administration of chorionic gonadotrophin to replace pregnant mare serum as soon as the maturation of the follicle is reflected by the fluctuations in the amount of cervical mucus."

Bereits 1934 wurde beobachtet, daß die Ovarien nur für einen begrenzten Zeitraum mit tierischen Gonadotropin-Präparaten stimulierbar waren. *J. C. Collip* gab als Erklärung für die nachlassende Wirkung die Bildung einer neuen Substanz, einem Anti-Hormon an, das die Wirkung der Gonadotropine verhindert (nach *Zondek* und *Sulman*, 1942). Damit war die Bildung von Antikörpern gegen tierische Gonadotropine beschrieben, lange bevor die immunologischen Prozesse bewiesen wurden (Østergaard, 1942, *Zondek* und *Sulman*, 1942, Østergaard und *Hamburger*, 1949). In Deutschland hat vor allem *Staemmler* umfangreiche klinisch-experimentelle Untersuchungen mit PMS durchgeführt (*Staemmler*, 1957, 1961, 1964).

Nachdem erkannt worden war, daß Extrakte oder Präparate tierischen Ursprungs in relativ kurzer Zeit zur Bildung von „Antihormonen" führen und so ihre Wirkung verlieren, mußte gefolgert werden, daß nur speziesgleiche Präparate eine brauchbare Alternative sind. *Gertrude van Wagenen* und *Miriam Elizabeth Simpson* zeigten, daß mit Extrakten aus Affenhypophysen wiederholt Ovulationen bei Rhesusaffen ausgelöst werden können (1957).

Knobil, Kostyo und *Greep* (1959) gelang die Ovulationsauslösung bei hypophysektomierten Rhesusaffen mit porcine FSH und hCG. „The evidence suggests that gradual stimulation of the follicles with small doses of FSH followed by large doses of hCG in a time span corresponding to the follicular phase of the menstrual cycle is most likely to result in ovulation."

1961 erscheint eine kritische Übersichtsarbeit mit 195 Literaturzitaten von *Herbert L. Kotz* und *Walter Herrmann* an der Yale University, New Haven: „A Review of the Endocrine Induction of Human Ovulation". Die Ur-

PRODUCTION OF OVULATION IN THE HYPOPHY-SECTOMIZED RHESUS MONKEY[1]

E. KNOBIL, J. L. KOSTYO[2] AND R. O. GREEP

Department of Physiology, Harvard Medical School and Biological Research Laboratory, Harvard School of Dental Medicine, Boston, Massachusetts

ABSTRACT

The experimental induction of ovulation in the hypophysectomized rhesus monkey is reported. This was produced by appropriate treatment with desiccated thyroid, porcine FSH and HCG during a time interval roughly equivalent to the follicular phase of the menstrual cycle.

Knobli, E., J. L. Kostyo, R. O. Greep: Production of ovulation in the hypophysectomized rhesus monkey: (© Endocrine Society) Endocrinology 65 (1959) 487–493.

sachen der widersprüchlichen Resultate der bis dahin möglichen Gonadotropintherapie werden analysiert. „Different criteria of case selection, unsatisfactory gonadotropic preparations, and variations in timing and dose of drug administration are in part responsible." Noch 1968 wird von *Swyer* und Mitarbeitern ein Gonadotrophin Stimulation Test of Ovarian Function mit PMS empfohlen. „We are not in a position to affirm that there would be similar responsiveness, or lack of it, to human gonadotrophin. However, at the upper and lower ends of the scale of response this certainly seems probable; in the intermediate range there might be room for doubt" (*G. I. M. Swyer* et al., 1968).

Pietro Donini (·1910 Fermignano/Pesaro) am Istituto Nazionale Farmacologico „Serono" in Rom berichtete 1949 über die Herstellung eines Gonadotropinpräparates aus dem Urin postmenopausaler Frauen: Pergonal. 1950 begannen Untersuchungen von *Bruno Lunenfeld* und *Rudi Borth* an der Frauenklinik in Genf bei *H. de Watteville* zur Gewinnung humaner Gonadotropine mit Hilfe der Kaolin-Absorptions-Technik mit dem Ziel, die Bildung von Anti-Hormonen zu vermeiden. Sie konnten zeigen, daß die Extrakte biologisch aktiv waren, indem sie die Spermatogenese bei hypophysektomierten pubertären Ratten induzierten (*Borth* et al., 1954). „We stated that human menopausal gonadotrophin extract (hMG) contains therefore FSH and ICSH (LH) in comparable amounts, a fact which opens up interesting therapeutic possibilities." In weiteren Experimenten konnten die gleichen Autoren bei weiblichen hypophysektomierten Ratten Ovulationen auslösen (*Borth* et al., 1957).

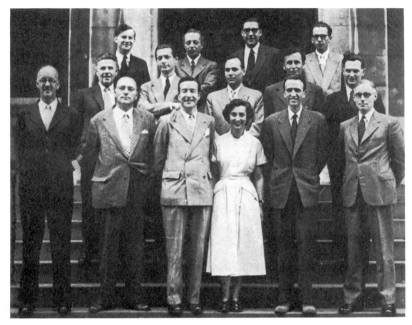

Plate 2.
Members of the 'G Club' Meeting in Birmingham, 1955. From left to right: front row: J. H. Gaddum, F. Benz, J. A. Loraine, Anita Mandl, R. Borth and A. C. Crooke. Middle row: J. Dekanski, E. Diczfalusy, B. Lunenfeld, J. B. Brown and W. R. Butt. Back row: P. S. Brown, S. Johnsen, A. A. Kinnear and K. Walter.

Club, G.: Birmingham 1955.

Im Sommer 1953 fand das erste Treffen des sog. G-Club in Genf statt, das zweite war 1955 in Birmingham. Vorwiegend wurden folgende Themen diskutiert: Assay-Methoden, Standards und Reinigungsmethoden zur Gewinnung therapeutisch einsetzbarer Präparate. Die erste Standard-Präparation wurde von *J. Dekansky,* Organon Newhouse in Schottland bereitgestellt: hMG 20. In einer kollaborativen Studie konnte die Brauchbarkeit dieses Präparates gezeigt werden (*Albert* et al., 1958). Der erste Internationale Standard für Serum-Gonadotropin (PMSG) wurde 1938 von der League of Nations eingeführt (League of Nations, 1938). 1961 veranlaßte das Expert Committee on Biological Standardization der WHO das National Institute for Medical Research in London einen zweiten Standard vorzubereiten. „In accordance with this authorization, the second International Standard for Serum Gonadotropin has been established with a potency of 1600 IU / ampoule. The International Unit for Serum Gonadotrophin is thus defined as the activity contained in 0.003569 mg of the second International Standard for Serum Gonadotrophin" (*Bangham* and *Woodward,* 1966). Das erste internationale Referenzpräparat für hMG wurde von *Donini* zur Verfügung gestellt und als solches 1974 von der WHO anerkannt (World Health Organisation, 1975). 1964 wurde der 2nd International Reference Preparation of Human Menopausal Gonadotrophins (FSH and LH), urinary for bioassay vom WHO Expert Committee on Biological Standardization mit 40 IU FSH und 40 IU LH pro Ampulle eingeführt. Der 1. Internationale Standard für urinäres FSH und für urinäres LH ersetzte 1976 die 2. IRP-HMG Reference Preparation (*Storring* et al., 1976). Auf Grund der Ergebnisse einer kollaborativen Studie enthielt eine Ampulle 54 IU FSH und 46 IU LH. Der 2. internationale Standard für human pituitary LH wurde 1992 eingeführt. Die Ampullen 80 / 552 enthalten 35 IU humanes LH (*Storring* und *Das,* 1993). Für hCG Immunoassays wurde 1980 ebenfalls vom National Institute for biological Standards, Holy Hill London ein Standard entwickelt (*Storring* et al., 1980). Dies geschah gleichzeitig auch für die α- und β-Subunits des hCG.

Die ersten hMG-Präparationen von *Donini* waren stark pyrogen. Nachdem weitere Reinigungen zu verträglicheren Chargen führten, konnte der klinische Einsatz beginnen. Im Dezember 1959 präsentierte *B. Lunenfeld* erste klinische Daten mit hMG in Gattlinburg. Mit hMG konnte eine Follikelreifung, aber noch keine Ovulation, induziert werden. Die Daten wurden 1961 publiziert (*Albert,* 1961). Die erste Publikation von *Lunenfeld, Menzi* und *Volet* in der eine Ovulationsauslösung durch Pergonal und hCG beschrieben wurde erschien 1960. Sie fanden einen erheblichen Anstieg der Östrogenausscheidung. Die erste Schwangerschaft und Geburt nach Ovulationsauslösung mit Pergonal war 1961 (*Lunenfeld* et al., 1962).

Carl Axel Gemzell (˙1910 Motala / Schweden) extrahierte als erster ein Präparat aus menschlichen Hypophysen und publizierte 1958 zusammen mit *Diczfalusy* und *Tillinger* die ersten klinischen Befunde mit diesem HP-FSH genannten Präparat. Die lyophilisierten Drüsen wurden mit CaO-Lösung extrahiert. Durch Präcipitation mit Ammoniumsulfat wurden die Gonadotropine ausgefällt, in Wasser gelöst, dialysiert und lyophilisiert. „Treatment with human pituitary FSH followed by HCG produced in all patients polycystic enlargement of the ovaries, ovulation in 4 out of 5, and a secretory transformation of the endometrium in 3 out of these 5 patients. Ovulation was accompanied by a marked incresae in the urinary excretion of both estrogen and pregnanediol." Auf dem Ciba-Symposium 1960 berichtet *Gemzell:* „It is apparent that HP-FSH is a potent hormone when tested in human beeings. In amenorrhoic women it produces enlarged polycystic ovaries and a great

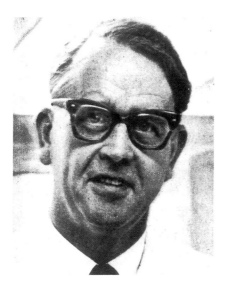

Gemzell, C.: 1910 Gynäkologe in Stockholm, Uppsala, New York. 1958 Clinical effect of human pituitary follicle-stimulating hormone (FSH). Zus. mit E. Dizcfalusy und K. G. Tillinger.

increase in urinary oestrogen. When HP-FSH was combined with the luteinizing factor in the form of hCG an ovulation occured and a corpus luteum was formed which was capable of secreting substantial amounts of progesterone as shown by the change of endometrium to secretory and by the greatly elevated output of pregnanediol. As shown in one case, the ova produced in this manner can be fertilized." *Gemzell* arbeitete von 1946 bis 1969 am Karolinska Hospital in Stockholm und von 1960 bis 1974 als Chairman in Uppsala.

C. L. Buxton und *W. Herrmann* (1961) in New Haven erprobten einen hypophysären Extrakt, der von Merck & Co zur Verfügung gestellt wurde. *Miriam Simpson* in Berkeley war verantwortlich für die Hypophysenpräparation und Austestung des Extraktes. Die lyophilisierten Hypophysen wurden mit 40% Ethanol extrahiert und mit höherer Alkoholkonzentration ausgefällt. Acht amenorrhoische Patientinnen wurden behandelt. „It would appear that the characteristic response following a full course of treatment is evidence of multiple ovulation. It is impossible to say, of course, whether these ovulations are otherwise normal, but it is possibly of some significance that non of our patients became pregnant and only 2 of *Gemzell's* patients have become pregnant to date so far as is known. Also of considerable significance is the fact that none of the patients who responded to therapy by menstruation and apparent ovulation continued to menstruate or ovulate subsequently." In einer zweiten Serie von 28 Zyklen bei elf Patientinnen mit

CLINICAL EFFECT OF HUMAN PITUITARY FOLLICLE-STIMULATING HORMONE (FSH)*

CARL A. GEMZELL, M.D., EGON DICZFALUSY, M.D. AND GUNNAR TILLINGER, M.D.

The Department of Obstetrics and Gynecology, Karolinska Hospital and King Gustaf V Research Institute, Stockholm, Sweden

ABSTRACT

A partially purified follicle-stimulating hormone preparation (human pituitary FSH) has been obtained from human pituitaries. The ovarian response to this preparation was studied in 7 amenorrheic women. The effect of human chorionic gonadotropin (HCG) was studied in addition.

In 4 patients exhibiting no endometrial activity or only slight proliferation, HCG alone did not induce ovulation and had no effect on the size of the uterus, on the endometrium, or on the urinary excretion of estrogen and pregnanediol. In 2 patients showing endometrial proliferation, the administration of HCG alone was followed by ovulation, a secretory transformation of the endometrium, and a marked increase in urinary pregnanediol excretion.

The administration of human pituitary FSH alone to 2 patients resulted in an increase in the size of the uterine cavity, in polycystic enlargement of the ovaries, and in a pronounced increase in urinary estrogen output.

Treatment with human pituitary FSH followed by HCG produced in all patients polycystic enlargement of the ovaries, ovulation in 4 out of 5, and a secretory transformation of the endometrium in 3 out of these 5 patients. Ovulation

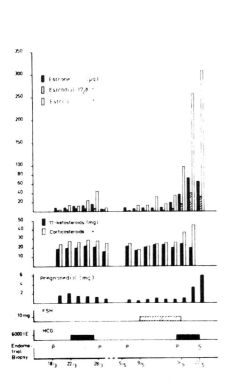

FIG. 5. Steroid excretion (48 hours) and endometrial activity in Case 4 during treatment with HCG and h.pit. FSH.

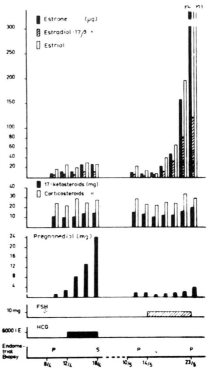

FIG. 6. Steroid excretion (48 hours) and endometrial activity in Case 5 during treatment with HCG and h.pit. FSH.

Gemzell, C., E. Diczfalusy, G. Tillinger: Clinical effect of human pituitary follicle-stimulating hormone (FSH). (© The Endocrine Society) J. Clin. Enedocrinol. 18 (1958) 1333–1348.

Induction of ovulation in the human with human gonadotropins

Preliminary report

C. LEE BUXTON, M.D.

WALTER HERRMANN, M.D.

New Haven, Connecticut

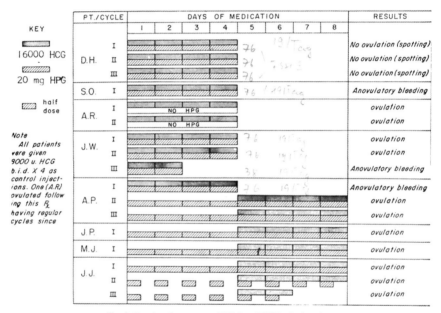

Fig. 1. Results of treatment (HCG and HPG) in 8 patients.

Buxton, C. L., W. Herrmann: Induction of ovulation in the human with human gonadotropins (permission granted Mosby Year Book) Am. J. Obst. & Gynec. 81 (1961) 584–590.

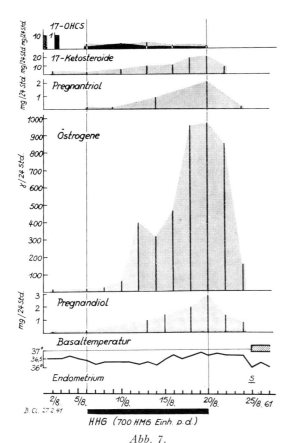

Apostolakis, M., G. Bettendorf, K. D. Voigt: Klinisch-experimentelle Studien mit menschlichem hypophysärem Hormon. Acta Endocrinol. 41 (1962) 14–30. (© European J. End. formerly Acta endocrin.).

Abb. 7.
Hormonausscheidung Pat. B. Cl., primäre Amenorrhoe.
Status nach Hypophysektomie   2. Behandlung

dem gleichen Extrakt weisen die Autoren auf die Bedeutung der FSH / LH-Relation hin. „... some combination of human gonadotropin containing FSH and LH is necessary to stimulate production of estrogen and progesterone by the ovary and, presumably, cause ovulation" (*Buxton, Kase, van Orden,* 1963).

In Hamburg wurde 1959 mit der Extraktion humaner Hypophysen begonnen. Die von *Koenig* und *King* (1950) beschriebene Methode mit ethanolischem Puffer führte zu einer guten Ausbeute und Anreicherung gonadotroper Aktivität (siehe S. 110). Das Präparat wurde hypophysäres Human Gonadotropin (hHG) genannt, da es sowohl FSH- als auch LH-Aktivität enthielt. Die ersten Klinischen Beobachtungen wurden 1961 in Wien vorge-tragen, in der gleichen Sitzung, in der *Lunenfeld* seine Befunde mit hMG berichtete (*Bettendorf,* 1961). Die erste Gravidität wurde 1962 erzielt (*Apo-stolakis, Bettendorf, Voigt,* 1962). Die Relation von FSH:LH war in den hHG-Extrakten nicht konstant. So ergab sich die Möglichkeit, den Einfluß der unterschiedlichen Aktivitäten auf die klinische Wirksamkeit zu überprü-fen. Es zeigte sich, daß Präparationen mit einem Quotient zwischen 0,05 und 10 von FSH:LH keinen wesentlichen Unterschied in ihrer Wirksamkeit aufwiesen (*Bettendorf* et al., 1968). „Man hat jedoch den Eindruck, daß Prä-parate mit einer FSH/LH-Relation zwischen 0,3 und 1,0 optimaler sind als solche mit niedrigeren oder höheren Relationen. Betrachten wir die Bezie-hungen der Überreaktionen zu der FSH/LH-Ratio, dann findet man die kleinste Zahl der Überstimulierungen in der Gruppe mit einem Quotienten von 0,3–1" (*Bettendorf* et al., 1970). Mit einer differenzierten Extraktion wurde eine Fraktion mit hoher LH-Aktivität gewonnen, mit der Ovulationen ausgelöst werden konnten (*Breckwoldt* et al., 1967).

M. Simpson und *G. von Wagenen* konnten bei Affen mit hMG Ovulatio-nen mit und ohne zusätzliche hCG-Gabe auslösen. *Jeanette McArthur* nann-te die Methode zur Kontrolle der Ovarreaktion „by means of a bioassay wit-hin the patient". Bei Stimulationen bei präpuberalen Tieren fand sich in der Regel ein Corpus luteum, dagegen bei erwachsenen immer multiple Ovula-tionen mit zwei bis elf Corpora lutea. Beim Vergleich der effektiven Dosis von Schaf-Gonadotropin mit Affen-Gonadotropin zeigte sich, daß von letz-terem 1/10 der Dosis wirksam war (1962).

Es erwies sich die individuell angepaßte Dosierung von hMG als vorteil-haft: „. . . monitored by a combination of chemical and clinical indices adju-sted to the requirements of the individual animal, dependably induced single ovulation" (*J. Ovadia* et al., 1971, *J. McArthur,* 1973). Diese Erfahrung be-stätigte sich auch in der klinischen Anwendung.

M. Breckwoldt untersuchte die Wirkung verschiedener Gonadotropin-Präparate bei Rhesus-Affen. „These findings may indicate that a certain amount of LH is required to bring the follicle to full maturity" (*Breckwoldt* u. *Bettendorf,* 1970).

Von besonderem Interesse war die Ovulationsauslösung bei hypophysek-tomierten Frauen, bei denen bis dahin keine Möglichkeit bestand schwanger zu werden. 1963 konnte die erste Schwangerschaft bei einer total hypophys-ektomierten Frau in Hamburg nach Ovulationsauslösung mit hMG erzielt werden (*Bettendorf,* 1963, *Bettendorf, Breckwoldt, Knörr, Stegner,* 1964). In der 31. Woche kam es zur Frühgeburt von Zwillingen. Die zweite Behand-

Tabelle.   *FSH und LH-Aktivität/mg verschiedener Gonadotropinpräparate aus menschlichen Hypophysen bzw. Urin*

(Augmentationstest gegen NIH-FSH S1. Ascorbinsäuretest gegen NIH-LH B1.)

Substanz	Untersucher	FSH (STEELMAN u. POHLEY) × NIH FSH S1	LH (PARLOW) × NIH-LH B1	FSH/ LH
Human L 581037-0-3 (STEELMAN, Merck Inst. Ther. Res.)	PARLOW u. REICHERT Endocrinology **73**, 740 (1963)	0,69	0,04	17,25
FSH Lot C-2023 (Merck & Co., Pens. USA)	ROSEMBERG et al. J. clin. Endocr. **24**, 105 (1964)	0,92		
FSH Lot C-2225 (Merck & Co., Pens. USA)	ROSEMBERG et al. J. clin. Endocr. **24**, 105 (1964)	0,97		
FSH (LI, San Francisco)	ROSEMBERG et al. J. clin. Endocr. **24**, 105 (1964)	0,97		
HP-FSH (Gemzell)	LINDELL, A., Acta endocrin. **47**, 277 (1964)	1,5		
HHG E_3 (BETTENDORF)	BETTENDORF et al. Acta endocr. **41**, 1 (1962); Arch. Gynäk. **199**, 423 (1964)	7,85 (3—15)	0,42 (0,02—1,4)	18,69
HHG $E_3 \times$ G 100	CZYGAN, P. J. et al. (1964)	21,8	0,5	43,6
a) Pergonal 22-C	ROSEMBERG et al. J. clin. Endocr. **24**, 105, 673 (1964)	0,32	0,20	1,60
b) Pergonal 25-EX-1899	ROSEMBERG et al. J. clin. Endocr. **24**, 105, 673 (1964)	1,44	0,28	5,14
NIH-FSH S1 (OVINE)	ROSEMBERG et al. J. clin. Endocr. **24**, 105, 673 (1964)	1,00	0,007	142,8

Breckwoldt, M., J. M. Angulo, G. Bettendorf: Follikelstimulierende und luteinisierende Aktivität verschiedener humaner Gonadotropinpräparate. (Vortrag 35. Tagung Deutsche Ges. Gyn. München 1964)Arch. Gyn. 202 (1964) 234–236.

Serien	Ausbeute von je 25 gR_1	FSH-NiH-S_3 Augmentations Test	LH-NiH-B_3 (OAAD)	FSH/LH	FSH* IE	LH* IE	FSH/LH
N_4 A65	44,5 mg	2,5	1,4	1,79	66,5	2153	0,03
N_4 B65	15,8 mg	>0,1	0,15	0,66	>2,6	230	>0,01
N_4 C65	45,3 mg	0,31	0,27	1,12	8,25	415	0,02
N_4 D65	142,2 mg	0,88	0,23	3,82	23,4	353	0,06
N_4 F65	16,3 mg	0,34	0,41	0,83	9,0	630	0,01
N_4 A65	174,0 mg	0,61	0,27	2,26	16,2	415	0,03

Abb. 86
Spezifische Aktivität menschlicher hypophysärer LH-Präparate (die Testung erfolgte gegen die NIH-Standards).

* Die Aktivitäten wurden nach *Reichert und Parlow (1964)* in Internationale Einheiten umgerechnet.

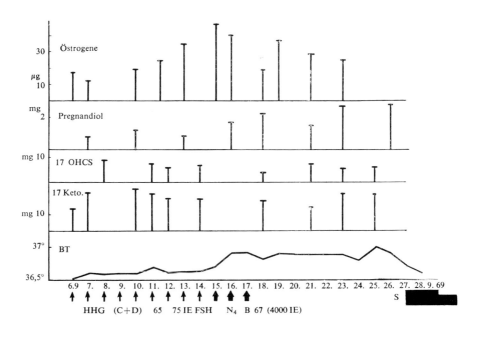

Abb. 87
Pat. I.H. sekundäre eugonadotrope Amenorrhoe. Reaktion auf die Verabreichung von
HHG und HLH

Breckwoldt, M., In Louwrens, B.: Menschliche Gonadotropine. Acta Endocrinol. Suppl. 148 (1970) 103 (permission granted European J. of Endocrinol., formerly Acta Endocrinol.). Rundtischgespräch, Tel-Hashomer, Israel, Mai 1968.

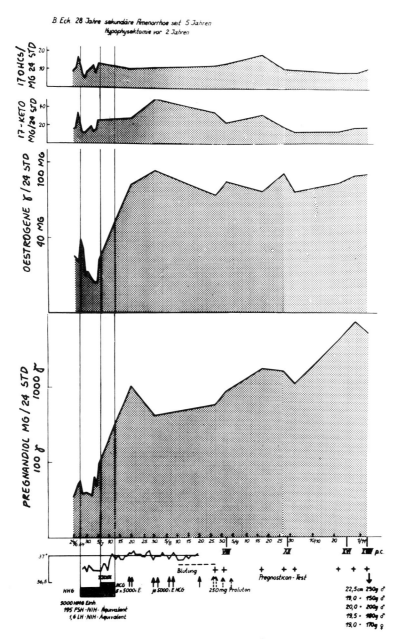

Fig. 5. Patient B. Eck., 28 years. Hormone excretion during the second HHG treatment with subsequent pregnancy and abortion of quintuplets in the 19th week.

Bettendorf, G.: Ovarian Stimulation in hypophysectomized Patients by Human Gonadotropins. V. World Congr. on Fertility and Sterility, Stockholm, Juni 1966.

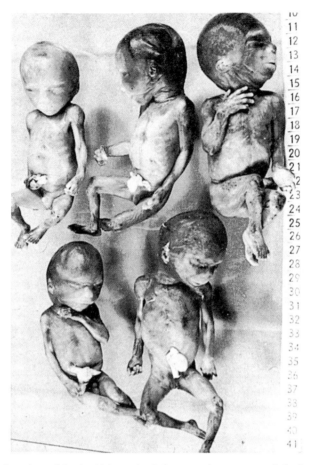

Fig. 4. Quintuplets aborted in the 19th week of the second pregnancy of the hypophysectomized patient (B. Eck.).

Bettendorf, G.: Ovarian Stimulation in hypophysectomized Patients by Human Gonadotropins. V. World Congr. on Fertility and Sterility, Stockholm, Juni 1966.

lung führte bei der gleichen Patientin zu einer Fünflingsgravidität, die in der 19. Woche lebensfrisch geboren wurden, aber nicht überlebten. Beim dritten Versuch resultierte eine Einlingsschwangerschaft mit Geburt eines gesunden Jungen. Bei dieser Patientin und weiteren hypophysektomierten mit völliger Funktionsruhe der Ovarien zeigte sich, daß die Therapiekontrolle einfacher war als bei Patienten mit partiell gestörter Funktion. Diese Beobachtung führte später zur Entwicklung des pharmakologisch induzierten Hypogonadotropismus mit LH-RH-Analoga (*Bettendorf* et al., 1981). Von *T. Luukainen* und *H. Adlerkreutz* in Helsinki wurden die Plasmasulfat-konjugierten Steroide, sowie im Urin Pregnandiol, Ketosteroide und elf Östrogene der hypophysektomierten Patienten analysiert (*Luukainen* et al., 1970). *Corral*, *Calderon* und *Goldzieher* waren der Meinung, daß sie die erste Gravidität bei einem Status nach Hypophysektomie durch eine hMG-Behandlung beobachtet hätten (*Corral* et al., 1972). *Gemzell* berichtet 1973 über fünf Frauen nach Operation von Hypophysen-Adenomen. „Four of the women conceived; three grave birth to twins and one to a single infant. The seven children were normal and healthy." Eine Zusammenstellung der Schwangerschaftsverläufe bei Frauen mit einem Hypophysenadenom wurde von *Gemzell* 1979 erstellt und ein Protokoll zur Therapie vorgeschlagen (*Gemzell* u. *Wang*, 1979).

Zahlreiche Beobachtungen über den Verlauf nach einer Hypophysektomie, während einer Gravidität bei Tieren, wurden publiziert. *P. E. Smith* berichtete 1954 erstmalig über entsprechende Studien bei Affen. „The results of the complete removal of the intrasellar components of the hypophysis (hypophysectomy) in 20 pregnant rhesus monkeys are reported. The hypophysectomies were done between the 27th and 156th day after conception ±2 or in some cases 3 days. Ten of the animals went to term. Six living babies were delivered, in 2 cases by caesarean section. Of the 4 nonliving babies, 2 with breech presentations died during the birth, and 2 were stillborn after posthypophysectomy periods in excess of 30 days. The length of gestation was normal except in one case. Lactation was of brief duration. . . . Five animals aborted 23 to 58 days after hypophysectomy. In one the time of abortion was not definitely determined. Two operated upon on days 66 and 101 of pregnancy abortet within a week, and 2 operated upon on days 142 and 156 had stillbirth after 10 and 4 days, respectively."

Bei einer Patientin mit metastasierendem Mamma-Karzinom wurde in der 26. Woche eine Hypophysektomie durchgeführt. In der 35. Woche wurde die Geburt wegen einer Plazentainsuffizienz eingeleitet. Die Laktation kam nicht in Gang. Infolge einer Pneumonitis verstarb die Patientin 12 Tage post partum (*Little, Smith, Jessiman* et al., 1958).

Wegen eines chromophoben Adenoms wurde eine Patientin in der 12. Woche operiert. Unter der Substitution mit Hydrokortison, Schilddrüsenpulver und Vasopressin verlief die Schwangerschaft normal. Die Hormonausscheidung entsprach der Norm (Aldosteron, Pregnanediol, Pregnantriol, Estrogene, Gonadotropine). Die Laktation war minimal (*N. M. Kaplan*, 1961).

Für eine Anwendung der Gonadotropintherapie auf breiterer Basis war es fraglich, ob post mortem Hypophysen in genügender Zahl als Ausgangsmaterial zur Verfügung stehen würden. *Lunenfeld* 1963: „The scarcity of postmortem human pituitary glands (required for the production of this preparation) eliminates the possibilities of its widescale use" und *Gemzell* 1964: „It might be argued that due to scarcity of human pituitaries the treatment will be of theoretical rather than practical importance. This need to be so because it is not impossible to obtain human pituitaries and prepare the hormone from them. About 10 pituitaries are necessary for one ovulation and in general conception will take place. The FSH material can be most usefully employed if patients are carefully selected before treatment." In den Therapiezentren Uppsala, Birmingham und Hamburg wurden Hypophysenpräparate noch bis Mitte der 60er Jahre eingesetzt. Die Industrie extrahierte dagegen ausschließlich Menopausenurin, Serono in Rom Pergonal und Organon in Oss, Holland Humegon. Lediglich in Australien wurde die Präparation der Australien pituitary agency noch weiter zur Therapie verwandt. Von dort kamen dann auch die ersten Beobachtungen einer Creutzfeld-Jakob-Erkrankung nach Gonadotropin-Therapie (*Cochius* et al., 1990, *Dumble* und *Klein*, 1992).

Zwischen 1960 und 1970 wurde die Gonadotropin-Therapie zur etablierten Methode der Ovarialstimulation. Zahlreiche unterschiedliche Therapieschemata wurden angewendet. HMG stand in Ampullen zu 75 i. E. zur Verfügung. Meist wurde mit ein bis zwei Ampullen begonnen. Bei dem Dosis-fixierten Vorgehen wurde die Dosis bis zur hCG-Injektion beibehalten. Der Zeitpunkt der hCG-Verabreichung wurde von unterschiedlichen Parametern abhängig gemacht. Diese spiegeln die methodischen Entwicklungen wider. Zunächst wurden nur die klinischen Befunde herangezogen, die einen Hinweis auf eine ausreichende Östrogenbildung gaben: Palpation der Ovarien, Karyopyknose Index, Zervixsekret. Quantitativ genauer ließ sich diese durch die direkte Bestimmung der Östrogene durch die, von *J. B. Brown* (1968) entwickelte, fluorometrische Methode erfassen. Die Angaben über

„Idealwerte" lagen zwischen 50 und 150 μg. Schließlich wurde die Follikel-größe, sichtbar und meßbar im Ultraschall, als Kriterium herangezogen. Die Durchmesser entsprachen denen in Spontanzyklen. Zur Ovulationszeit fanden sich Werte von 17 bis 22 mm. Eine zeitliche und individuelle Zuordnung für die Einführung der verschiedenen Parameter ist kaum möglich. Nahezu zeitgleich wurden die Methoden in den wenigen Arbeitsgruppen zu dieser Zeit erprobt und in unterschiedlich großen Patienten-Kollektiven überprüft (Übersicht bei *Brown*, 1986, *Bettendorf,* 1989).

Bei den Dosis-fixierten Therapieschemata wurde die gleiche Dosis verabreicht, bis der gewünschte Effekt erreicht war oder eine bestimmte Dosis wurde an bestimmten Tagen gegeben. In Birmingham versuchten *Arthur C. Crooke* (˙1905 Frodingham, Lincolnshire – † 1990 Cherryholme/Kidderminster) und *Wilfried Butt* (˙ 1922 Souhthampton) die individuelle effektive Dosis zu ermitteln. Hypophysäres Gonadotropin wurde zusammen mit hCG als Einzelinjektion verabreicht an Tag 1, 4 und 8 und eine hCG-Injektion an Tag 10 (*Crooke* et al., 1963, *Crooke* et al., 1965). In einer weiteren Versuchsgruppe wurde neun Frauen eine einmalige Dosis FSH mit hCG und sieben bis neun Tage später eine zweite hCG-Injektion verabreicht. Diese Behandlung wurde alle drei Wochen wiederholt, bis ein positiver Respons, gemessen an der Östriol- und Pregnandiolausscheidung, eintrat. Diese Dosis war dann die effektive (*Crooke* et al., 1966). Dieses Vorgehen wurde modifiziert, indem eine FSH-Dosis allein an Tag 1 und hCG an Tag 9 oder 10 verabreicht wurden (*Crooke* et al., 1967). Schließlich überprüften die gleichen Autoren ein Schema mit zwei Injektionen pro Woche (*Crooke* et al., 1971). Bei all diesen Studien handelte es sich jedoch um kleine Patientenzahlen und zudem wurden hypophysäre und urinäre Präparate eingesetzt. 1970 berichteten *Crooke* und Mitarbeiter über bis dahin insgesamt 106 Frauen, die behandelt wurden, 44 wurden schwanger. Sechs Mehrlingsgraviditäten (Drillinge und mehr) traten ein. „Treatment with FSH which contained little LH was associated with few pregnancies with triplets or more but with more abortions than were those with FSH rich in LH" (*Crooke* et al., 1970).

Taymor beschrieb die step down Methode, „This approach should keep unwanted ovarian stimulation to a minimum" (*Taymor* et al., 1967).

Von den vielfältigen Therapieschemen erwies sich das „Threshold Dose Principle" als das beste Vorgehen. Es hatte sich gezeigt, daß die jeweilige Reaktion individuell von Patientin zu Patientin unterschiedlich war und ebenso in verschiedenen Zyklen der gleichen Patientin. Beginnend mit einer niedrigen Dosierung, wird diese stufenweise erhöht, bis eine Ovarialreaktion zu erkennen ist, d.h. die Schwellendosis erreicht ist (*Lunenfeld*, 1963, *Townsend*

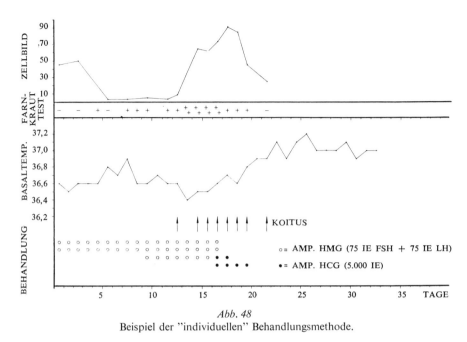

Abb. 48
Beispiel der "individuellen" Behandlungsmethode.

Insler, V., B. Lunenfeld: Das individuell angepaßte Behandlungsschema. In Louwrens, B.: Acta Endocrinol. Suppl. 148 (1970) 79 u. 85 (permission granted European J. of Endocrinol. formerly Acta Endocrinol) Rundtischgespräch, Tel-Hashomer, Israel, Mai 1968.

et al., 1966, *Bettendorf,* 1968). Die Mitteilungen gerieten offensichtlich in Vergessenheit und das gleiche Vorgehen wurde als „individual adjusted step-up regimen" oder „low dose" Therapie 20 Jahre später erneut beschrieben (*Seibel* et al., 1984; *Buvat* et al., 1989; *Meldrum* et al., 1991).

Einhergehend mit der neuen Möglichkeit eine ruhende Ovarialfunktion therapeutisch zu beeinflussen, ergab sich die Möglichkeit und die Notwendigkeit einer sachgemäßen Klassifikation ovarieller Funktionsstörungen. Die bisherigen Diagnosen basierten auf dem jeweiligen Hauptsymptom. Die unterschiedlichen Reaktionen auf die Gonadotropintherapie ermöglichten eine therapieorientierte Klassifikation. Als Parameter für eine entsprechende Klassifizierung erwies sich der Gonadotropin- und Östrogenstatus. Eine Einteilung nach diesen Werten wurde erstmals 1968 von *Vaclav Insler* und *Lunenfeld* auf einem Workshop in Tel-Hashomer vorgeschlagen (in *Louwrens,* 1970). Die Bezeichnung „hypo, normo, und hypergonadotrop" wurde eingeführt und erste Daten über die Bedeutung der FSH/LH-Relation vorgelegt (*Bettendorf* in *Louwrens,* 1970). Präparationen mit einer Relation um

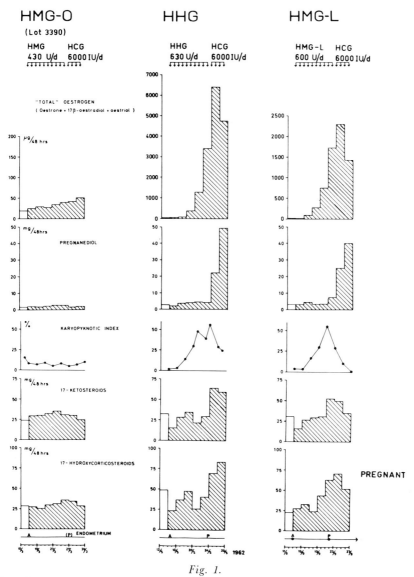

Fig. 1.

Clinical and steroid metabolic effects of various human gonadotrophins in a patient with secondary amenorrhoea (B. W. 28 years). HMG-O and HMG-L indicate human menopausal gonadotrophin preparations from Organon Ltd., Oss and AB Leo, Hälsingborg, respectively. HHG is a human hypophysial gonadotrophin and HCG a human chorionic gonadotrophin preparation. In each experiment open bars indicate the results of urinary steroid analyses prior to the administration of gonadotrophins. The amount of HMG or HHG activity administered is expressed in units per day (U/d) of the International Reference Preparation (I. R. P.) as assayed by the mouse uterine weight method. For the Follicle Stimulating Hormone (FSH) and Interstitial Cell Stimulating Hormone (ICSH) activities of the various preparations the data of Tables 5 and 6 should be consulted. For the purposes of the present investigation 1.0 unit of I. R. P. was defined as the gonadotrophic activity of 1.0 mg of I. R. P.

Diczfalusy, E., E. Johannison, K. G. Tillinger, G. Bettendorf: Comparison of the clinical and steroid metabolic effect of human pituitary and urinary gonadotrophins in amenorrhoic women. Acta Endorcinologica Suppl. 90 (1964) 35–56) (permission granted European J. of Endocrinology, formerly Acta Endocrinologica).

PERGONAL (MENOTROPINS): A SUMMARY OF CLINICAL EXPERIENCE IN THE INDUCTION OF OVULATION AND PREGNANCY

CHARLES R. THOMPSON, M.A., AND LAURA M. HANSEN, B.S.

Cutter Laboratories, Inc., Berkeley, California

TABLE 2. *Summary of Clinical Results with Menotropins Therapy in Patients with Various Diagnoses*

	Primary amenorrhea	Secondary amenorrhea	Secondary amenorrhea with galac- torrhea	Polycystic + probable polycystic ovaries	Anovulatory cycle, irregu- lar menses	Miscellaneous
Total no. patients	74	293	70	212	315	229
Total no. treatment courses	257	624	173	546	652	459
Ovulation						
Patients	46 (62%)	180 (61%)	54 (77%)	162 (76%)	243 (77%)	191 (83%)
Courses	97 (38%)	352 (56%)	92 (53%)	341 (62%)	438 (67%)	386 (84%)
Pregnancy attempted						
Patients	54	261	67	196	313	208
Courses	156	580	169	524	649	432
Pregnancy achieved						
Patients	12 (22%)	73 (28%)	28 (42%)	50 (26%)	76 (24%)	42 (20%)
Courses	14 (9%)	87 (15%)	33 (20%)	54 (10%)	81 (12%)	44 (10%)
Births	10	55	22	25	51	27
Abortions	2 (14%)	21 (24%)	7 (21%)	21 (39%)	12 (15%)	16 (36%)
Multiple pregnancies	3 (25%)	21 (28%)	12 (41%)	8 (17%)	9 (14%)	1 (2%)
2 concepti	3 (25%)	14 (18%)	9 (31%)	8 (17%)	6 (9%)	1 (2%)
3 or more concepti	0	7 (10%)	3 (10%)	0	3 (5%)	0
Fetal abnormalities	1 (8%)	0	1 (3%)	0	1 (2%)	2 (4.6%)
Still gravid	2	11	4	8	18	1
Hyperstimulation syndrome						
Courses	0	12 (1.9%)	2 (1.2%)	6 (1.1%)	13 (2.0%)	3 (0.7%)

Thompson, C., R. Hansen, L. M. Pergonal (menotropins): A summary of clinical experience in the induction of ovulation and pregnancy. Fertil. Sterlin. 21 (1970) 844–853. Reproduced with permission of the publisher, the American Society for Reproductive Medicine (formerly The American Fertility Society).

eins erwiesen sich als optimal. Vergleiche zwischen urinären Präparaten (hMG) und hypophysären (hHG oder HP-FSH) ergaben keine prinzipiellen Unterschiede. Die Ovarreaktion war abhängig von der verabreichten FSH-Aktivität. „The clinical effectiness of the various gonadotrophin preparations was found to be a function of the amount of FSH – rather than total gonadotrophic activity administered" (*Diczfalusy* et al., 1964).

Die Ergebnisse einer Gonadotropinbehandlung waren in den wenigen Arbeitsgruppen zu Anfang im wesentlichen gleich. So faßten *Gemzell* und *Roos* 1966 wie folgt zusammen: „During a 4 year period about 100 women with primary or secondary amenorrhea were treated for sterility with human pituitary FSH and HCG. About 90% ovulated once or several times, and

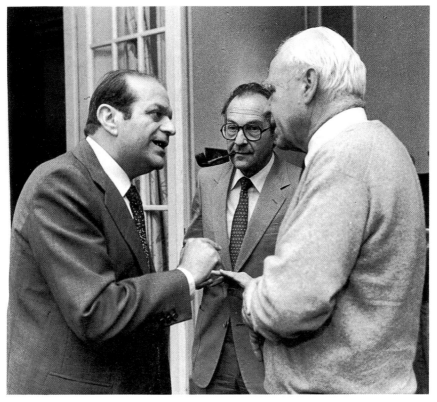

Insler, V., G. Bettendorf, G. Weiland (Organon): Auf dem Symposium Advances in Diagnosis and Treatment of Infertility 1980 in Bad Reichenhall. *Günter Weiland* war von 1966 bis 1985 Geschäftsführer der Organon in München, er ermöglichte die Organon Symposien und hat durch seine vielseitigen Aktivitäten wesentlich zur Entwicklung der Endokrinologie beigetragen.

50% became pregnant. So far 43 have been delivered, 20 women of a single infant, 14 of twins, and 9 of triplets or more fetuses. Thus, the incidence of multible births was the same as that of single births. Repeated pregnancies were induced in 10 patients. The rate of abortion was high in those women who conceived triplets or more while it was negligible in those with single pregnancies. No congenital malformations were observed. To avoid multiple births the daily dose of human pituitary FSH, the pattern of FSH administration and the endogenous gonadotropin production must be taken into careful consideration with each new patient. This kind of treatment is, therefore, best confined to special centers with a fully equipped gynecologic endocrine unit" (*Gemzell* and *Roos,* 1966).

Eine Übersicht über die gepoolten Ergebnisse von 100 Untersuchern in den USA und Kanada stammt von *Thompson* und *Hansen* (1970). Es wurden 1286 Patienten in 3002 Zyklen behandelt. Die Schwangerschaftsrate war 25 %, Aborte 25 %, und schwere Überstimulation 1,3 %. „The treatment schedule of choice was daily administration of menotropins for 9–12 days, followed by administration of 6000–10 000 IU of HCG 1 or 2 days after the last menotropins injection. ... The ovulation rate was similar in all diagnostic groups, ranging from 61–83 %." Die Verabreichung von LH-RH anstelle von hCG führte ebenfalls zu Ovulationen (*Breckwoldt* et al., 1974), wie auch das von *Donini* hergestellte desialo-hCG (*Bettendorf* u. *Leidenberger*, 1976).

Es erscheint wichtig auf die damaligen Möglichkeiten zum Nachweis einer Ovarialreaktion hinzuweisen. Als Maß für die Follikelfunktion dient die Östrogenproduktion. Chemische Bestimmungen der Östrogenausscheidung waren sehr aufwendig und konnten wegen des über mehrere Tage gehenden Verfahrens nicht zur aktuellen Kontrolle benutzt werden. In den ersten Jahren wurde der Effekt einer Gonadotropin-Stimulation auch durch direkte Inspektion der Ovarien bei einer Laparoskopie oder Laparotomie überprüft. Als Beweis für eine induzierte Ovulation diente der histologische Nachweis einer sekretorischen Umwandlung des Endometriums und ein Anstieg der Basaltemperatur. Biologischer Parameter für eine Veränderung der Östrogenaktivität war der Vaginal-Abstrich. Der Karyopyknose-Index zeigte eine gute Korrelation zu den Östrogenwerten. Das Zervixsekret wurde erst in den 60er Jahren als guter und einfach zu erfassender Parameter erkannt. *Vaclav Insler* (* 1929 in Stanislawow / Polen) kommt der Verdienst zu für die Östrogenwirkung den Zervixindex (Insler Score) vorgeschlagen zu haben. „According to this method, the amount, spinnbarkeit and ferning of the cervical mucus and the appearance of the external cervical os are estimated and each parameter is given a score of 0–3. The sum of scores given to individual parameters represents the combined Cervical Score" (*Insler* in *Bettendorf* u. *Insler* 1970 und *Insler* et al., 1973). Ein großer Fortschritt war die Entwicklung einer Methode, mit der Östrogene schnell und zuverlässig gemessen werden konnten. *Brown* beschrieb 1968 die halb-automatische fluormetrische Methode zur Messung des Gesamtöstrogens im Harn, die zehn bis zwölf Bestimmungen in vier Stunden ermöglichte (*J. B. Brown*, 1968). 1977 wurden systematische Untersuchungen zur sonographischen Kontrolle des Follikelwachstums von *Hackeloer* vorgelegt (*Hackeloer* et al., 1977). Bald konnte die Bedeutung dieses Verfahrens für die Therapiekontrolle bewiesen werden (*Hackeloer* et al., 1980, *Nitschke-Dabelstein* et al., 1980).

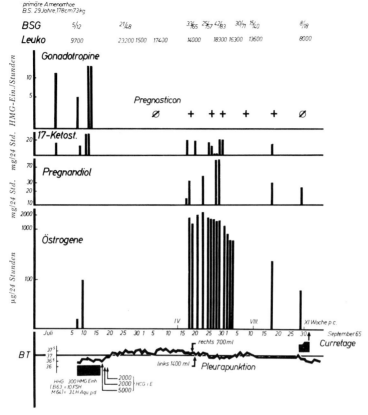

Abb. 1 Pat. B. S., 29 Jahre, primäre eugonadotrope Amenorrhoe. Hormonanalysen während der HHG-Therapie und der nachfolgenden Gravidität.

Bettendorf, G., D. Ahrens, K. Groot, J.-H. Napp: Akutes Meigs- Syndrom und Gravidität nach Ovulationsauslösung mit hypophysärem Human- Gonadotropin. Geburtsh. Frauenheilkd. 26 (1966) 1281–1287.

Lunenfeld berichtete im Juni 1980 auf einem Workshop in Bad Reichenhall über die gepoolten Daten von 914 Patienten mit 2890 Behandlungszyklen der vergangenen 20 Jahre. Die Schwangerschaftsrate in Gruppe I, d.h. bei hypogonadotropen Patienten war 84%, bei Gruppe II, d.h. Patienten mit normalen Gonadotropinwerten und vorhandener Östrogenaktivität 21%. Die Abortrate lag bei 23%, die Mehrlingsinzidenz bei 28,79%. In 3% wurde eine leichte Überstimulierung beobachtet, in 0,28% eine schwere (*Lunenfeld* et al., 1981).

In der gleichen Sitzung wurden die Hamburger Ergebnisse vorgetragen. 765 Frauen wurden in 1585 Zyklen behandelt. Es resultierten 239 Gravidi-

Laboratoriums- und klinische Befunde			Unerwünschte		Neben-erscheinungen	
			leicht		schwer	
	I	II	III	IV	V	VI
Östrogene > 150 ug/24 St.	+	+	+	+	+	+
Pregnandiol > 10 mg/24 St.	+	+	+	+	+	+
Vergrösserte Ovarien		+	+	+	+	+
Palpable Zysten		?	+	+	+	+
Auftreibung des Abdomens			+	+	+	+
Schwindel			+	+	+	+
Erbrechen				+	+	+
Durchfall				?	+	+
Aszites					+	+
Hydrothorax					?	+
Veränderungen des Blut-volumens, der Viskosität und der Koagulationszeit						+
	erfordert keine Behandlung		erfordert Beobachtung		erfordert Krankenhaus-aufnahme	

Insler, V.: Klassifizierung der Hyperstimulierung. In Louwrens, B. 1968 (85) (Abb. 52).

täten (33%) (*Bettendorf* et al., 1981). Die Ergebnisse in den verschiedenen Diagnostik-Gruppen waren unterschiedlich. Patientinnen mit anovulatorischem Zyklus oder mit einer Corpus luteum-Insuffizienz, die nicht auf Clomiphen reagiert hatten, zeigten auch nach hMG schlechtere Resultate. Zugleich ergab sich eine prozentuelle Zunahme dieser Gruppe im Beobachtungszeitraum. „The more severe the gonadotropin stimulation defect, the better the chance for the patient to conceive during gonadotrophin therapy" (*Bettendorf* et al., 1981). Aufgrund dieser Beobachtung wurde der Effekt einer Stimulation bei gleichzeitiger Blockade der endogenen Hypophysenfunktion überprüft und später das Therapiekonzept der Vorbehandlung mit LHRH-Analoga entwickelt (*Fleming*, 1982, *Bettendorf* et al., 1981). Die Ursache für die Diskrepanz zwischen Ovulations- und Schwangerschaftsrate wurde vor allem von *F. Lehmann* (1978) in seiner umfangreichen Habilitationsarbeit auf die häufig zu beobachtende Insuffizienz der Lutealphase zurückgeführt. *C. J. Kubik* zitierte acht Jahre später die Arbeit von *Olson* et al. (1983). „The data in this paper are the first to show any evidence of shortened luteal phases following hMG-stimulated cycles" (*Kubik*, 1986). Ein klassisches Beispiel dafür wie wenig sorgfältig die Ergebnisse anderer registriert werden. *J. B. Brown* (1986) stellte die Resultate der mit hPG behandelten 243 Frauen zusammen. Aus 262 Schwangerschaften resultierten, 21 % Mehrlinge, 18 % Aborte. Die Dosierung erfolgte aufgrund der Ergebnisse eines Gonadotropin-Stimulation-Tests. An drei Tagen wurde je 150 iE FSH verabreicht. Ein Östrogenanstieg an Tag 3 und 6 diente als positiver Respons. Bei negativem Ergebnis wurde die Dosis verdoppelt. Die aktuelle Behandlungsdosis war zwei Drittel der Dosis mit der eine positive Reaktion beobachtet wurde.

Die Rate der kongenitalen Fehlbildungen nach Stimulation war nicht erhöht (*Hack* et al., 1970, *Caspi* et al., 1976, *Zimmermann* et al., 1981, 1982). Auch Langzeituntersuchungen der Kinder ergaben keine Auffälligkeiten, vor allem war das Karzinomrisiko nicht erhöht (*Lunenfeld* et al., 1981, *Lunenfeld* and *Lunenfeld*, 1988).

Eine besondere Herausforderung war die unphysiologische Reaktion der Ovarien mit der Folge von Polyovulationen, Überstimulierungen und Mehrlingsschwangerschaften. Die Analyse der ovariellen Steroide ergab eine im Vergleich zum Normalzyklus gesteigerte Östrogen- und Progesteronproduktion (*Taymor*, 1968, *J. B. Brown* et al., 1969, *Bettendorf* et al., 1972, *Czygan*, 1974). Die Häufigkeit von Mehrlingen lag zwischen zehn und 40 % (*Gemzell* und *Roos*, 1966, *Schenker* et al., 1981, *Zimmermann* et al., 1982, *J. B. Brown*, 1986). Das gefürchtete Ovar-Hyperstimulations-Syndrom (OHS) wurde bereits bei der PMS-Therapie beobachtet (*Staemmler*, 1964). Mit unterschiedlicher Häufigkeit wird diese Komplikation in allen Studien in Abhängigkeit von der Zahl und der Zusammensetzung des Patientenguts aufgeführt. Die erste schwere Überstimulation mit Todesfolge beschrieb 1958 *Figuera-Cases*. Das klinische Bild mit Ausbildung eines Aszites und Hydrothorax, das akute *Meigs* Syndrom, wurde 1965 erstmals beobachtet (*Bettendorf* et al., 1965, *Neuwirth* et al., 1965). *Meigs* und *Cass* hatten 1937 die Symptomenkombination Ovarialfibrom mit Hydrothorax und Aszites beschrieben. Vereinzelt kam es zur Ruptur oder zur Stieldrehung der polyzystisch vergrößerten Ovarien, wodurch eine Laparotomie erforderlich wurde (*Neuwirth* et al., 1965, *Bettendorf*, 1965). Die Einteilung der Klinik des OHS in drei Schweregrade erfolgte 1967 durch *Rabau*. Über die Pathophysiologie konnten keine eindeutigen Aussagen gemacht werden (*Bettendorf* u. *Lindner*, 1987). Da die Überstimulation mit einer erhöhten Kapillarpermeabilität einhergeht, wurde die Hypothese aufgestellt, daß ovarielle Substanzen im Übermaß gebildet einen kapillaren Flüssigkeitsverlust verursachen (*Polishuk* und *Schenker*, 1969). Sowohl Histamin (*Knox*, 1974), als auch Prolaktin

(*Leung* et al., 1983) und Prostaglandine (*Pride* et al., 1984) wurden diskutiert. Die Hyperviskosität des Blutes mit pathologisch erhöhten Gerinnungsparametern kann zu schweren thromboembolischen Ereignissen führen (*Philipps* et al., 1975). Es wurden Amputationen und Todesfälle beobachtet (*Moses* et al., 1965). Eine Einschränkung der Nierenfunktion führt zu einer Erhöhung harnpflichtiger Substanzen (*Engel* et al., 1972).

Auf dem WHO-Workshop 1973 über „Agents stimulating gonadal function in the human" konnten die wesentlichen Aspekte im Hinblick auf Patientenselektion, Dosierung, Kontrolle der Therapie und Nebenwirkungen zusammengefaßt werden.

Die I. therapieorientierte WHO-Klassifikation der Ovarialinsuffizienz wurde aufgrund des Gonadotropin Status erarbeitet. 1975 erfolgte in einer WHO Sitzung in Hamburg eine Erweiterung durch Hinzuziehung des Prolactin als zusätzlichem Parameter: II. WHO Klassifikation.

Eshkol und *Lunenfeld* beobachteten 1967, daß gereinigte FSH-Präparate bei juvenilen Mäusen ein Follikelwachstum induzieren ohne daß es zu einer Östrogenbildung kommt (*Eshkol* u. *Lunenfeld,* 1967). *Donini* fand, daß FSH ohne LH kein Uteruswachstum induziert und daß ein Dosis abhängiges Uteruswachstum mit steigendem LH-Zusatz resultiert (*Donini* et al., 1970).

Die Ergebnisse der klinischen Anwendung des von *Donini* hergestellten, gereinigten, urinärem FSH (Metrodin) waren nicht einheitlich. Einige Untersucher fanden bessere Resultate mit dem „reinen" FSH beim PCO (*Braendle* et al., 1981, *Venturoli* et al., 1982, 1983). *Birkhäuser* (1988) wies auf die mögliche Bedeutung „überflüssiger" LH-Aktivität hin. Von ihm stammt auch die größte Gruppe, die mit Metrodin behandelt wurde. Bei 40 Patienten resultierten in 89 Zyklen 23 Schwangerschaften (57,5 %) (*Birkhäuser,* 1991). *Claman* und *Seibel* (1986) stellten die Ergebnisse von 10 Autoren zusammen. Nach Therapie mit gereinigtem FSH wurden bei 88 Patienten in 156 Zyklen 99 Ovulationen induziert und 32 Graviditäten erzielt.

Inzwischen steht ein wesentlich reineres Präparat im rekombinanten FSH zur Verfügung. Die Expression von humanem FSHdimer konnte in Hamster-Ovarien mit einem genomischen Klon der kompletten FSH β-kodierenden Sequenz zusammen mit einem α-Subunit Minigen erzielt werden. Pharmakologische Untersuchungen wurden durchgeführt (*le Cotonnec* et al., 1994, *Hornnes* et al., 1993, *Matikainen* et al., 1994). Erste klinische Untersuchungen haben zu Ovulationen und Schwangerschaften geführt (*Devroey* et al., 1992, 1993, *Germond* et al., 1992).

Das Auftreten der Creutzfeldt-Jakob'schen Erkrankung nach einer Therapie mit hypophysären Gonadotropin-Extrakten war, anders als nach einer

WHO SCIENTIFIC GROUP ON AGENTS STIMULATING GONADAL FUNCTION IN THE HUMAN

Geneva, 28 August - 1 September 1972

Members:

Professor Gerhard Bettendorf, Department of Obstetrics and Gynaecology, University of Hamburg, Federal Republic of Germany

Professor J. Ferin, Department of Obstetrics and Gynaecology, University of Louvain, Belgium

Professor C. Gemzell, Department of Obstetrics and Gynaecology, University Hospital, Uppsala, Sweden (*Vice-Chairman*)

Dr R. Greenblatt, Department of Endocrinology, Medical College of Georgia, Augusta, Ga., USA

Dr C. Gual, Chairman, Research Division, Department of Endocrinology, National Institute of Nutrition, Mexico D.F., Mexico

Professor B. Lunenfeld, Director, Institute of Endocrinology, The Sheba Medical Centre, Tel Hashomer Government Hospital, Israel (*Chairman*)

Professor S. Matsumoto, Department of Obstetrics and Gynaecology, School of Medicine, Gunma University, Maebashi, Japan

Professor C.A. Paulsen, Department of Medicine, School of Medicine, University of Washington, Seattle, Wash., USA (*Rapporteur*)

Representatives of other organizations:

International Federation of Gynecology and Obstetrics:

Professor H. de Watteville, Secretary General, International Federation of Gynecology and Obstetrics, Geneva, Switzerland

Secretariat:

Professor E. Diczfalusy, Director, Reproductive Endocrinology Research Unit, Karolinska Hospital, Stockholm, Sweden (*Temporary Adviser*)

Dr A. Kessler, Chief, Human Reproduction, WHO, Geneva, Switzerland (*Secretary*)

Dr I. Manuilova, Chairman of Obstetrics and Gynaecology, First Medical Institute, Moscow, USSR (*Temporary Adviser*)

WHO Agents stimulating gonadal function in the human. WHO techn. Rep. Ser. 1973, No 514.

hGH-Therapie, auf Einzelfälle begrenzt (*Cochius* et al., 1990, *Dumble* u. *Klein*, 1992).

Das Anliegen der klassischen Gonadotropintherapie war eine möglichst dem physiologischen Ablauf entsprechende Ovarstimulation zu erzielen. Dies konnte mit der individuell angepaßten Dosierung annäherungsweise erreicht werden. Die Methoden der assistierten Reproduktion, wie IVF und GIFT führten dazu, daß man möglichst mehrere Eizellen zur Fertilisation haben wollte. Folge davon war die Rückkehr zu einer Schematisierung der Therapie mit festgelegter Dosierung. Dies führte beim Einsatz zur „in vivo" Fertilisation zu einer erneuten Zunahme von unerwünschten Überstimulationen. Als Folge davon wurde das niedrig dosierte, individuell angepaßte Vorgehen wieder neu entdeckt und propagiert (*Seibel*, 1984, *Buvat*, 1989, *Meldrum*, 1991).

Die Behandlung des männlichen Hypogonadismus wurde vergleichsweise nur gering durch den Einsatz humaner Gonadotropine beeinflußt. Eine Stimulation der Spermiogenese in hypophysektomierten Männern wurde von *McLeod* (1964, 1966) berichtet. Die Hodenbiopsie 100 Tage nach Therapiebeginn zeigte eine komplette Spermiogenese, aber keine Leydigzellproliferation. Die Testosteronwerte blieben niedrig und es kam nicht zu Ejakulationen. *Mancini* (1969) bewirkte bei Hypophysektomierten mit hCG eine Stimulation der Sertolizellen, eine Ausreifung des Germinalepithels, und eine Proliferation der Leydigzellen. Die Kombination von hMG mit hCG verstärkte die Wirkung von hMG. Gleichzeitige Testosterongabe hatte einen hemmenden Effekt. *Gemzell* und *Kjessler* (1964) erzielten bei partiell hypophysektomierten Männern mit hPG nach 13 Wochen eine Spermiogenese. Zwei von *Lunenfeld* behandelte Männer waren in der Lage Kinder zu zeugen (1978). Gute Resultate wurden bei der Therapie von Patienten mit einem hypogonadotropen Hypogonadismus erzielt (*Heller*, 1965, *Davies*, 1965, *Johnsen*, 1966, *Paulsen*, 1965).

Nach *Lunenfeld* et al. (1979) reagieren Männer mit einer Oligospermie nur dann, wenn niedrige FSH-Werte vorliegen und die FSH-Reaktion auf GnRH erniedrigt ist. In einer Plazebo-kontrollierten, Doppelblind Studie fanden *Knuth* et al. (1987) keinen Effekt auf die Spermienkonzentration bei Oligospermie.

Entwicklung der Gonadotropin-Forschung im Spiegel der Symposien und Workshops

Zur Intensivierung der Gonadotropin-Forschung und zum jeweils aktuellen Informationsaustausch haben die Kleinkonferenzen wesentlich beigetragen. Der meist familiäre Geist der Zusammenkünfte der zahlenmäßig kleinen Gruppe, war für den wissenschaftlichen Fortschritt von Bedeutung. Die erste Tagung des „G-Clubs" wurde 1954 von *de Watteville* in Genf organisiert. Teilnehmer waren: *A. C. Crooke* und *W. Butt* aus Birmingham, *J. B. Brown* und *J. Loraine* aus Edinburgh und *B. Lunenfeld* und *R. Borth* aus Genf. Weitere Treffen des G-Clubs folgten 1955 in Birmingham, 1957 in London, 1961 in Kopenhagen und 1966 in Edinburgh. Die Endocrinology Study Section regte die „Workshop-conference on assays for hormones" an, die 1959 unter Leitung von *A. Albert* in Gatlinburg/Tennessee stattfand. 28 aktive Teilnehmer wurden eingeladen. *Emil Witschi* war der Organisator der Tagung der Ford Foundation „The Physiology of Reproduction" 1966 in Venedig. 1968 fand in der Royal Society of Medicin in London die Konferenz „Developments of the pharmacology and clinical use of human gonadotropin" statt. Im Anschluß an den VI. World Congress on Fertility and Sterility im Mai 1968 in Tel-Aviv traf man sich in Tel-Hashomer. Nur vier Wochen später war ein von *Eugenia Rosemberg* organisierter Workshop in Vista Hermosa, vor dem internationalen Endokrinologenkongreß in Mexico-City. Hier wurde zum erstenmal über den Einsatz der Isoelektrofokussierung bei der Reinigung der Gonadotropine berichtet (*Bettendorf* et al., *Saxena* et al.). 1969 leiteten *Crooke* und *Butt* in Birmingham die Tagung „Gonadotropins and ovarian development". Unter der Schirmherrschaft der WHO fand eine Workshop-Konferenz mit dem Titel „Clinical application of human gonadotropins" in Hamburg statt. Sponsor dieser Tagung waren die Firmen Organon, die das hMG-Präparat Humegon produzierten und Merck, die in Deutschland zu der Zeit das Pergonal der Serono vertrieben. Im Oktober 1970 initiierte *Frederick Zuspan*, Chicago ein Symposium „Treatment of the infertile female: Ovulation stimulating drugs". Anläßlich der 200. Jahrestagung der Society of the New York Hospital organisierten *Fuchs, Peterson, Sa-*

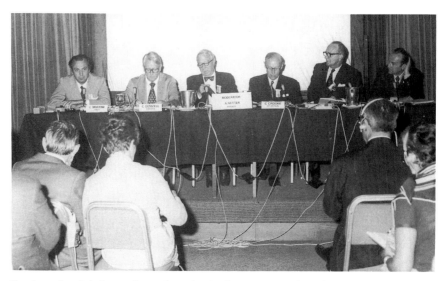

Panel on the clinical use of gonadotropins in the treatment of sterility in women. V. World Congr. of Fertility and Sterility, Stockholm 1966 (von li.: L. Martini, C. Gemzell, A. Netter, C. Crooke, H. de Watteville, G. Bettendorf).

xena, Gandy und Behling ein Symposium in der Cornell University. Tibor Klacansky aus Bratislava machte es möglich in der Zeit des kalten Krieges in der hohen Tatra ein Treffen durchzuführen: „Symposium on Gonadotropins in Endocrine Disorder of Human Reproduction". Richtungweisend wurde die Task force Sitzung der WHO-Scientific Group on agent stimulating gonadal function in the human 1972 in Genf. Übereinstimmung wurde erzielt über eine Klassifikation der Ovarialinsuffizienz auf der Grundlage des Gonadotropinstatus, Kriterien für das Monitoring einer Stimulationstherapie wurden festgelegt und die Wertigkeit verschiedener Stimulationsprotokolle diskutiert. Unter der Leitung von Meinert Breckwoldt war 1975 in Freiburg ein Serono-Symposium „Ovulation in the Human". Eine Revision und Erweiterung der 1. WHO-Klassifikation der Ovarialinsuffizienz erfolgte auf der 2. Sitzung der WHO-Scientific Group im Juli 1975 in Hamburg. Als zusätzlicher Parameter zum Östrogen- und Gonadotropinstatus wurde der Prolaktinwert herangezogen. Im November 1976 war das WHO-Symposium „Regulation of Human Fertility" unter der Leitung von Egon Diczfalusy in Moskau. Ein weiteres Organon-Symposium ermöglichte Günter Weiland im Juli 1980 in Bad Reichenhall: „Advances in Diagnosis and Treatment of Infertility". Im November 1980 war in San Marino das Serono-Symposium „The

Gonadotropins, basic sciences and clinical aspects in females", im Juni 1982 das Organon-Symposium „Fertilisation of the human egg in vitro" in Bad Reichenhall. Im September 1985 wurde in Hamburg auf einer Kleinkonferenz die Frage diskutiert, ob ein Unterschied besteht bei einer Ovarialstimulation für eine in-vivo im Vergleich zur in-vitro Befruchtung. 1986 im Mai wurden ebenfalls in Hamburg Aspekte der Wissenschaftsgeschichte der Gonadotropine in Chemie, Biologie und Reproduktionsmedizin behandelt. *M. Breckwoldt* führte im April 1989 in Freiburg und *Frank Lehmann* im August 1989 in Bielefeld das Symposium „Gonadotropine, Drei Jahrzehnte Entwicklung – HMG-Behandlung in der Praxis" durch.

Die wichtigsten Etappen in Kürze

Die Erforschung der Hypophysenvorderlappenhormone begann zu Anfang unseres Jahrhunderts. Die Ergebnisse klinischer Beobachtungen und tierexperimenteller Untersuchungen wurden zur Grundlage des Wissens. Bis 1935 war der Nachweis der drei Gonadotropine FSH, LH und hCG erbracht, die physiologischen Funktionen und ansatzweise auch die klinischen Folgerungen erforscht. In der Zeit danach wurden Versuche zur Reindarstellung unternommen, biologische Nachweismethoden wurden entwickelt und mit diesen Ausscheidungsprofile erstellt. Bereits in den 30er Jahren begann der klinische-therapeutische Einsatz von Extrakten, Implantaten und Hormonpräparationen. Mit dem Einsatz homologer Präparate wurde erstmals eine gezielte Stimulation der Gonaden möglich. Der Aufschwung in der Reproduktionsmedizin ist weitgehend hierauf zurückzuführen. Der Einsatz neuer chemischer Verfahren ermöglichte die Aufklärung der chemischen Struktur. Mit den immunologischen Methoden wurde der Nachweis hormoneller Aktivität wesentlich genauer und leichter. Hierdurch konnten die Kenntnisse über die Physiologie und Pathophysiologie der Gonadotropine erweitert werden. Die Bedeutung des Polymorphismus ist noch nicht geklärt. Die Erprobung gentechnisch hergestellter FSH-Präparate eröffnet ein neues Kapitel der Gonadotropinforschung.

Prolaktin

Auf die Arbeiten von *Halban* (1905) über den Einfluß der Plazenta auf die Laktation wurde bereits hingewiesen. Eine Wirkung der Hypophyse auf die Laktation beschrieb 1915 *Walter Lee Gaines*. *P. Stricker* und *F. Grüter* in Straßburg machten die Beobachtung, daß bei ovariektomierten pseudograviden Kaninchen durch Extrakte vom Hypophysenvorderlappen eine Laktation bewirkt wird, aber nicht bei unreifen Tieren (*Stricker* und *Grüter*, 1928, 1929). Den gleichen Effekt fanden sie auch bei Hunden, Kühen und Schweinen. *Evans* und *Simpson* (1930) konnten mit alkalischen Extrakten bei virginellen Ratten Brustwachstum und Laktation induzieren. *G. W. Corner* (1930) zeigte, daß auch ovariektomierte Tiere entsprechend reagierten.

John Hunter hatte 1786 „pigeons milk" entdeckt, eine Substanz, die von beiden Elterntieren vom Kropf zum Füttern der jungen Tauben sezerniert wird. Etwa 150 Jahre später fanden *Riddle* und Mitarbeiter, daß dieser Kropfsackeffekt unter der Kontrolle der Adenohypophyse steht (*Riddle* et al., 1931, 1932). *Oscar Riddle*, *Robert W. Bates* und *S. W. Dykshorn* publizierten 1933 ihre Befunde zur „Preparation, identification and assay of prolactin – a hormone of the anterior pituitary". In *Riddles* Arbeiten werden die Arbeiten von *Stricker* und *Grüter* nicht zitiert, die beiden Forscher hätten nicht den Nachweis eines eigenständigen Prolaktins erbracht. Er beanspruchte für sich und *Bates*, Prolaktin entdeckt zu haben (*Riddle*, 1955). Sie gaben dem Hormon auch den Namen Prolaktin. *Charles W. Turner* hatte den Namen Galaktin oder Lactogen benutzt, *William R. Lyons* Mammotropin.

Die Arbeitsgruppe in Chicago fand auch den Einfluß von Prolaktin auf das Brutverhalten von Hühnern und das mütterliche Verhalten von Ratten (*Riddle* et al., 1935). Der Ausdruck „mother-love-hormone" wurde geprägt. *Noble* et al. (1936) induzierten Brutverhalten bei Fischen. Die Kontrolle der Corpus luteum-Funktion bei Ratten durch Prolaktin wurde von *Astwood* (1941) und von *Evans* et al. (1941) entdeckt. Aufgrund dieser Wirkung wurde der Name Luteotropin geprägt. Eine Beschreibung der vergleichenden Physiologie findet man bei *Bern* und *Nicoll* (1968).

Die chemische Struktur von ovinem Prolaktin wurde von *Cho Haoh Li* aufgeklärt (*Li*, 1961, 1972, *Li* et al., 1969). Es fand sich eine Peptidkette mit 198 Aminosäuren mit einem Molekulargewicht von 23 000. *Li* führte die laktogene Aktivität von Primatenhypophysen auf die Wirkung von Wachstumshormon zurück. *Friesen* zeigte jedoch, daß auch bei Primaten Prolaktin ein eigenständiges Hormon ist und entwickelte eine RIA für humanes Prolaktin (*Hwang* et al., 1971, *Friesen* et al., 1971, 1972, 1974). *Niswender* et al. hatten 1969 einen RIA für Ratten Prolaktin publiziert. Die komplette Aminosäuresequenz wurde von *Shome* und *Parlow* bestimmt (1977). Die Möglichkeit das Hormon zu messen und die Einführung des Dopaminagonisten Bromocriptin (*E. Flückiger* et al., 1972, *del Pozo* et al., 1972), dem ersten Prolaktininhibitor, waren die Voraussetzungen für die weitere Aufklärung der Physiologie und Pathologie des Prolaktin. Die physiologische Funktion von Prolaktin wurde von *Werner O. Nelson* und *Joseph Meites* bearbeitet (*Meites*, 1988).

Wachstumshormon

Herbert M. Evans und *J. A. Long* zeigten 1921, daß die Injektion von Vorderlappenextrakt über drei Monate bei Ratten das Wachstum stimuliert. Wurde die Behandlung über neun Monate fortgesetzt, resultierte ein Gigantismus. Die Tiere erreichten ein Gewicht von 900 g und waren zweimal so groß wie normale erwachsene Tiere (*Evans* und *Long*, 1922). *Philip E. Smith* erzielte bei hypophysektomierten Tieren mit frischem Hypophysengewebe eine völlige Normalisierung des Wachstums (1930). Als Ausgangsmaterial für die weitere Reinigung diente ein alkalischer Gewebsextrakt (*Evans* et al., 1933). Als Bio-Assay wurde die Wirkung des Hormons auf die Tibiaepiphysenfuge entwickelt, der Tibiatest (*Evans* et al., 1943). In den 60er Jahren wurde der RIA für STH eingeführt (*Utiger* et al., 1962). 1944–45 wurde von *Li, Miriam Simpson* und *Evans* die Isolierung von bovinem Wachstumshormon berichtet. *Wilhelmi, Fishman* und *Russel* erzielten 1948 mit einer alkoholischen Extraktion eine bessere Ausbeute und eine kristalline Präparation. Die chemische und physikochemische Charakterisierung erfolgte in Berkeley (*Li*, 1957, *Papkoff* et al., 1962) und ebenfalls die Strukturaufklärung (*Li* et al., 1971, 1972), gleichzeitig auch durch *Santomé* et al. (1971). Von *Li* wurde die Bezeichnung „Somatotropin" vorgeschlagen, da das Hormon neben dem Wachstumseffekt zahlreiche andere Wirkungen besitzt (*Li*, 1957).

Evans berichtete 1935 über klinische Versuche beim menschlichen Zwergwuchs: „...has been treated with pituitary extracts by several careful workers who have reported that children who had ceased growth or were growing at a subnormal rate, resumed normal growth or even exceeded the growth rate normal for the age at treatment" (*Evans*, 1935). *Knobil* und *Greep* (1959) verabreichten homologes Hormon hypophysektomierten Affen und beobachteten eine Stickstoffretention, ein Knochenwachstum und eine Normalisierung des Kohlenhydratstoffwechsels. *Beck* und Mitarbeiter wiesen eine Wirkung von humanem Hormon und von Affen-Hormon beim Menschen nach (1957). *M. S. Raben* behandelte erstmals 1958 einen hypophysären Zwerg mit humanem Wachstumshormon. Der klinische Einsatz führte zur Aufklärung der Stoffwechselwirkungen (*Prader,* 1965, *Schönberg* u. *Bierich,* 1966, *Illig* et al., 1969).

Gravierend war die Beobachtung, daß bei Patienten, die mit extrahiertem hGH behandelt wurden, später eine Creutzfeldt-Jakob'sche Erkrankung auftrat. So kam die Aufklärung der primären Struktur des humanen Gens zur Kodierung für hGH Ende der 70er Jahre zum richtigen Zeitpunkt (*Seeburg* et al., 1977, *Martial* et al., 1979). Dies war die Voraussetzung zur Herstellung von rekombinanten hGH. Seit 1981 wird anstelle der aus Extrakten gewonnenen Präparate nur noch das rekombinante hGH klinisch eingesetzt.

Thyroidea-Stimulierendes Hormon (TSH)

1851 beobachtete *B. Niepce* in Paris die Vergrößerung der Hypophyse in Verbindung mit einer parenchymatösen Struma. Ein funktioneller Zusammenhang wurde aber nicht erkannt. Zwei Jahre vorher hatte *Berthold* in Göttingen seine klassischen Experimente zum Nachweis einer hormonellen, durch das Blut vermittelten Wirkung publiziert (1849). *Sir William Gull* verknüpfte die Symptome beim Myxödem mit einer Atrophie der Schilddrüse (1874). Die Brüder *Reverdin* entfernten die Schilddrüse zur Behandlung der Struma und stellten fest, daß die Patienten myxödematös wurden (1883, zitiert nach *Greep*, 1974). Der Einfluß der Hypophyse auf die Schilddrüse nach Hypophysektomie wurde von *Aschner* (1912), *Adler* (1914), *P. E. Smith* (1916), *B. M. Allen* (1916) untersucht. Vorderlappenextrakte führten zur Normalisierung der Schilddrüsenfunktion. *Anderson* und *Collip* beschrieben eine Hyperplasie und einen Hyperthyreoidismus bei hypophysektomierten Ratten nach partiell gereinigtem TSH (1932). Der erste qualitative Bioassay, von *Junkmann* und *Schoeller* entwickelt, basierte auf den histologischen Veränderungen in Meerschweinchen-Schilddrüsen (1932). Zwischen 1930 und 1950 wurden Extraktions- und Reinigungsverfahren entwickelt die zu einer Aktivitätsanreicherung führten. Es ergab sich, daß die Trennung von TSH und LH die Isolierung erschwerte. Die Reinigung mittels Ionen-Austausch-Chromatographie führte zu höheren Aktivitäten, und es fanden sich multiple aktive Formen. Ebenso wie bei FSH und LH erwies sich TSH auch als ein Glykoprotein. Zudem zeigten LH und TSH viele Gemeinsamkeiten. Nachdem für LH die Subunit-Struktur entdeckt war, fand man diese auch beim TSH (*Pierce*, 1974).

Adrenocorticotropes Hormon (ACTH)

R. *Zander* beschrieb 1890 eine Beziehung zwischen Nebennierenrinde und anderen Organen, vor allem dem Großhirn. Er bezog sich dabei auf frühere Berichte über die Befunde bei Anencephalen.

Eine adrenale Atrophie nach Hypophysektomie bei Hunden wurde 1912 von *Ascoli* und *Legnani* beobachtet. *Morris Simmonds* äußerte sich bei der Diskussion in seiner Arbeit „Atrophie des Hypophysenvorderlappens und hypophysäre Kachexie" 1918 folgendermaßen: „Daß es sich um eine primäre Schädigung des Hirnanhangs handelt, an die sich sekundär die Veränderungen der Schilddrüse, Nebenniere und Genitalien anschließen: Damit wird aber die nahe Verwandtschaft zwischen multipler Blutdrüsennekrose und Vorderlappenatrophie mit hypophysärer Kachexie zugegeben." Ein Jahr später berichtete *Hofstätter* (1919) über die Verdopplung des adrenalen Gewebes nach Hypophysenextrakten beim Hund. *P. E. Smith* machte bei Ratten ähnliche Beobachtungen, eine Atrophie nach Hypophysektomie und eine Reversion durch Hypophysenextrakte (*Smith*, 1926, 1927, 1930). Aufgrund der großen Löslichkeit von ACTH, überrascht es nicht, daß mit Wachstumshormon- und Prolaktinextrakten Effekte an der Nebennierenrinde gefunden wurden. Den ersten gesicherten Nachweis einer adrenokortikotropen Wirkung verdanken wir *James Bertram Collip* zusammen mit *E. M. Anderson* und *D. L. Thomson* in Toronto. Sie isolierten 1933 ein „adrenotrophin" Hormon durch isoelektrische Präzipitation. Das reine ACTH wurde zehn Jahre später in Berkeley von *Li, Simpson* und *Evans* aus Schafs-Hypophysen gewonnen und von *Georg Sayers, A. White* und *C. N. H. Long* in Yale aus Schweine-Drüsen (1943). *Sayers* Arbeitsgruppe entwickelten den Cholesterondepletionstest (1943) und den Ascorbinsäuredepletionstest (1944). *Philip Showalter Hench* verdanken wir den Nachweis der Wirkung von Rindenhormonen und von ACTH beim Rheumatismus (*Hench* et al., 1949). Die Aminosäuresequenz des bovinen ACTH wurde von *Li* et al. (1961) und des humanen von *Lee* et al. (1961) aufgeklärt. Die Polypeptide-Kette besteht aus 39 Aminosäuren mit einem Molekulargewicht von 4500. Speziesunterschiede finden sich in Position 25 bis 33, die aber nicht für die biologische Aktivität von Bedeutung sind. Die Synthese der aktiven Peptide gelang *Hofmann* und Mitarbeiter 1962 und die Totalsynthese von Schweine-ACTH 1963 *Schwyzer* und *Sieber.*

Ein starker Anstieg von Plasma-ACTH findet sich nach totaler beidseitiger Adrenalektomie, wenn sich ein chromophobes Adenom entwickelt: Nelson Syndrom (*Nelson* et al., 1960).

Melanonzytenstimulierendes Hormon (MSH)

Die Existenz eines Stoffes in der Hypophyse, der ein Dunkelwerden der Haut bei Fröschen und Kaulquappen hervorruft, wurde von *Smith* (1916) und *B. M. Allen* (1916) entdeckt. Gereinigtes MSH wurde aus Hypophysen von Schwein, Rind, Pferd und Affen gewonnen. Schweine-MSH enthält α- und β-MSH. Die Peptidkette ist identisch mit der von ACTH in den N-terminalen 13 Aminosäuren (*K. Hofmann,* 1974). α-MSH ist ein 13 Aminosäuren-Peptid. β-MSH hat 22 Aminosäuren. Das α-Peptid wurde in menschlichen Hypophysen nicht gefunden. MSH bewirkt Melanindispersion bei Reptilien. Bei Mammalien spielt es eine Rolle beim saisonalen Farbwechsel in der Haut. Bei Menschen bewirkt es ein dunkler werden der Haut (*Novales,* 1974). Die Injektion von synthetischem MSH führt bei Männern zu einem LH- und FSH-Anstieg (*Reid* et al., 1981). Die physiologische Bedeutung beim Menschen ist unklar. β-Lipotropin wurde von *Li* 1964 aus Rinder- und Schweine-Hypophysen isoliert. *Cseh* et al. (1972) und *Scott* und *Lowry* (1974) reinigten menschliches β-LPH. Das Peptid besteht aus 91 Aminsäuren mit einem Molekulargewicht von 11 700 (*Li* und *Chung,* 1976). Die Peptidhormone ACTH, Lipotropin und die Endorphine sind Spaltprodukte von einem gemeinsamen Precursor, einem Glykopeptid mit einem Molekulargewicht von 31 000 (*Odell,* 1979). Die Physiologie ist nicht bekannt. *Chretien* und *Li* postulierten eine Rolle als Prohormon für β-MSH, dessen Sequenz der von β-LPH 41−58 entpricht (*Chretien,* 1973). In Hypophysenschnitten wurde die Biosynthese von β-LPH nachgewiesen und die Transformation in β-Endorphin (β-LPH 61−91), gamma-LPH 1−58 und β-MSH (βLPH 41−58) (*Chretien* et al., 1976, zitiert nach *Bowers* et al., 1979).

Neurohypophyse

1895 berichteten *G. Oliver* und *E. A. Schäfer* in einer vorläufigen Mitteilung im Journal of Physiology, daß Extrakte von frischen Hypophysen nach intravenöser Injektion bei anästhesierten Tieren einen Blutdruckanstieg bewirkten. *W. H. Howell,* Physiologe an der Johns Hopkins Universität, konnte das Wirkungsprinzip im Hinterlappen lokalisieren (1898). Sowohl *Howell* (1898) als auch *Schäfer* und *Vincent* (1899) beobachteten einen Pressor- und einen Depressoreffekt von Extrakten. Die Reinigung der Neurohypophysen-Hormone war einfach im Vergleich zu denen der Adenohyophyse. Die biologischen Wirkungen konnten durch Blutdruckmessungen und Beobachtungen der Uteruskontraktionen erfaßt werden. *Sir Henry Dale* entdeckte 1906 die stimulierende Wirkung auf den Uterus. Dieser oxytocische Effekt wurde 1909 von *Hochwart* und *Fröhlich* in Wien bestätigt. Im gleichen Jahr setzte *Blair Bell* Hinterlappenextrakte klinisch ein. Er beobachtete bei Sectiones eine Uteruskontraktion (*Bell,* 1909). *Foges* und *Hofstätter* (1910) behandelten postpartale Blutungen mit „Pituitrin". *Hofbauer* (1911) und *Gottfried* (1911) testeten Extrakte bei Wehenschwäche.

Paulesco, Aschner und *Cushing* hatten bei ihren Experimenten gezeigt, daß die Entfernung des Hinterlappens keine fatalen Auswirkungen hat und keine Symptome hervorruft wie bei der Cachexia hypophysiopriva. *Percy Theodor Herring* in Edinburgh (1872–1967) beschrieb 1908 Kolloidtropfen im Hinterlappen. *Cushing* nahm an, daß es sich hierbei um Hormone handle (1910).

I. Ott, Physiologe in Philadelphia, und *J. C. Scott* (1910) berichteten über ein galaktokinetisches Prinzip in Hinterlappenextrakten, nachgewiesen bei Ziegen. *Schäfer* und *MacKenzie* bestätigten dies bei Hunden und Katzen (1911). *Edward Albert Schäfer* fand 1913, daß nicht die Milchproduktion gesteigert wird. *Heaney* (1913) injizierte Pituitrin laktierenden Frauen. Die Wirkung bestand nicht in einer Steigerung der Milchproduktion, sondern lediglich auf einer Beeinflussung der Muskelfasern. *Schäfer* (1850–1935) der

Sohn eines Hamburger Kaufmanns, war Physiologe in Edinburgh. Nach 1918 nannte er sich *Sharpey-Schafer.*

Neben der Wirkung auf die Gefäße beobachtete *Schäfer* auch eine Beeinflussung der Nierenfunktion (1908). Die antidiuretische Wirkung wurde 1915 von *A. Konschegg* und *E. Schuster* beschrieben. *F. von Hann* fand, daß beim Diabetes insipidus der Hinterlappen zerstört ist (1918). Die Ausdrücke Oxytozin und Vasopressin wurden von *O. Kamm,* der bei *Parke-Davis* in den USA arbeitete, geprägt (1928). Der Begriff Antidiuretin hat sich nicht durchgesetzt.

Die Analyse und die Synthese von Oxytozin und Vasopressin erfolgte zwischen 1953 und 1958 durch die Arbeitsgruppe von *V. du Vigneaud* (1953, 1958). Die Struktur von Arginin-Vasopressin wurde von der gleichen Gruppe und gleichzeitig von *Acher* und *Chauvet* aufgeklärt (1953). Lysin-Vasopressin hat die gleiche Sequenz, anstelle von Arginin findet sich Lysin (*du Vigneaud,* 1954). Die Synthese beider Vasopressine gelang auch der *Cornell*-Gruppe (*du Vigneaud,* 1954). *Van Dyke* et al. (1942) fanden ein hochmolekulares Peptid mit oxytocischer und vasopressorischer Aktivität. *Acher* und Mitarbeiter (1956) zeigten, daß die beiden Hormone an ein Trägerprotein Neurophysin gebunden sind.

Die Neurohypophysären Hormone wurden bei zahlreichen Spezies nachgewiesen (*Acher,* 1974). Eine Zusammenstellung der evolutionären Aspekte findet man bei *H. Heller* (1974) und bei *R. Acher* (1974).

Schlußbetrachtung

Versucht man eine Wertung der Forschungsabläufe, so waren die ersten 10–20 Jahre die, in denen mit den „einfachen" Mitteln der klassischen Endokrinologie die wesentlichen Grundlagen erarbeitet wurden. Die Originalität der Experimente dieser Pionierzeit kann nicht hoch genug eingestuft werden. Besonders hervorzuheben ist die Leistung einiger Wissenschaftler, die Pioniere der Erforschung der Hypophysen-Vorderlappen-Hormone waren: *Bernhard Aschner, Philip Edward Smith, Harvey W. Cushing, Herbert McLean Evans, Selmar Aschheim, Bernhard Zondek, Frederick Lee Hisaw, Cho Haoh Li.* Auf deren grundlegenden Arbeiten aufbauend konnten die Hypophysen-Hormone zur Diagnostik und zur Therapie in der Klinik eingesetzt werden und führten zu neuen Erkenntnissen über die Regulation und Funktion der Gonaden, der Schilddrüse und der Nebennierenrinde. Die Entwicklungen in der Reproduktionsmedizin sind ohne den Einsatz der Gonadotropine nicht denkbar. Sowohl ACTH, als auch STH und TSH wurden zu nicht mehr weg zu denkenden Faktoren in der klinischen Medizin. Die klassische endokrinologische Forschung geht zu Ende. Die Endokrinologie wird mit dem Einsatz molekularbiologischer Methoden eine neue Dimension bekommen. Zum Verständnis der mit diesen erzielten neuen Befunden ist aber das Wissen um die klassische Endokrinologie Voraussetzung.

Soweit ein geraffter Einblick in die Geschichte der hypophysären Hormone, der vielleicht anregt, einmal in nur 30, 50 oder 60 Jahren alten Publikationen zu lesen, vor allem, wenn man selbst auf diesem Gebiet arbeiten will und meint etwas Neues entdeckt zu haben. Die Zeitschriften sind voll von nicht originellen Wiederholungen. *J. B. Brown* schreibt: „At that time it was a crime not to have read every paper ever published on the subject before starting work, something which would be impossible today" (*J. B. Brown,* 1995).

„Du fragst, was Geschichte heißt?
Daß man beim Staffellauf den Stab zuverlässig weiterreicht."
(KoUn ‚Die Sterne über dem Land der Väter.' Suhrkamp 1996)

Literatur

A: Übersichten

Bahl, O. P.: The Chemistry and Biology of Human Chorionic Gonadotropins and its Subunits. In Greep, R., M. A. Koblinsky (eds.): Frontiers in Reproduction and Fertility Control. MIT Press Cambridge, Mass. and London, England (1977).

Bettendorf, G.: Historischer Überblick über die ersten 3 Jahrzehnte der Gonadotropin-Behandlung. In Lehmann, F., M. Breckwoldt: Gonadotropine, HMG-Behandlung in der Praxis. Bücherei des Frauenarztes, Band 39 (1991) 1–9.

Bettendorf, G.: Zur Geschichte der Endokrinologie und Reproduktionsmedizin, 256 Biographien und Berichte. Springer, Berlin, Heidelberg, New York (1995).

Chen, S. H., E. E. Wallach: Five decades of progress in management of the infertile couple. Fertil. Steril. 62 (1994) 665–685.

Engelhard, von D., F. Hartmann: Klassiker der Medizin I und II. Beck'sche Verlagsbuchh. München (1991).

Everett, J. W.: Pituitary and Hypothalamus: Perspectives and Overview. In Knobil, E., J. Neill et al. (eds.): The Physiology of Reproduction. Raven Press, Ltd. New York (1988) 1143–1159.

Greep, R. O.: The saga and the science of the gonadotrophins. The Sir Henry Dale Lecture for 1967. Proc. Soc. Endocrinol. II–IX (1967).

Greep, R. O.: History on research on anterior hypophysial hormones. In Greep, R. O., E. B. Astwood (eds.): Handbook of Physiology, Vol IV The Pituitary gland and its neuroendocrine control. Am. Physiol. Soc., Washington (1974) 1–27.

Greep, R. O.: Reproductive Endocrinology: Concepts and Perspectives, an Overview. Rec. Progr. Horm. Res. 34 (1978) 1–23.

Greep, R. O.: The gonadotrophins and their releasing factors. J. Reprod. Fert. Suppl. 20 (1973) 1–9.

Hamburger, Ch.: Historical Introduction. In Ciba Foundation Study Groups No 22: Gonadotropins, Physicochemical and Immunological Properties. J. A. Churchill, LTD, London (1965).

Karger-Decker, B.: An der Pforte des Lebens. Wegbereiter der Heilkunde im Portrait. Edition q, Berlin 1991.

Lehmann, F.: Untersuchungen zur menschlichen Corpus luteum Funktion. Grosse Verlag, Berlin (1978).

Lichtenthaeler, Ch.: Medizinhistorische Voraussetzungen zu einer Erneuerung in der Theorie der Medizin. J. F. Lehmanns, München (1963).

Lichtenthaeler, Ch.: Geschichte der Medizin. Deutscher Ärzte Verlag, Köln (1987 + 1988).

Meites, J., B. T. Donovan, S. M. McCann: Pioneers in Neuroendocrinology, New York Plenum (1975).

McCann, S. M.: Endocrinology, People and Ideas. Am. Phsiol. Soc. Bethesda Ma. (1988).

O'Dowd, M. J., E. E. Philipp: The History of Obstetrics and Gynecology. Parthenon Publ. Group, New York, London (1994).

Papkoff, H., R. J. Ryan, D. N. Ward: The Gonadotropic Hormones, LH (ICSH) and FSH. In Greep, R., M. A. Koblinsky (eds.): Frontiers in Reproduction and Fertility Control. The MIT Press, Cambridge, London (1977) 1–10.

Pappenberger, R.: Abhängigkeit der gonadalen Funktion vom zentralen Nervensystem. Inaugural-Dissertation, Erlangen, Nürnberg (1985).

Pierce, J. G.: Gonadotropins: Chemistry and Biosynthesis. In Knobil, E., J. Neill et al. (eds.): The Physiology of Reproduction. Raven Press, Ltd. New York (1988) 1335–1348.

Rolleston, H. D.: The endocrine organs in health and disease with an historical review. University Press, London, Oxford (1936).

Simmer, H. H., J. Süss: Östrogenforschung 1844–1948. Eine kommentierte Bibliographie, 3. Teil. IV. Hypophysenvorderlappen und Ovarien. Frühe Beobachtungen und Experimente. Gynäkol. u. Geburtsh. 16, 323–328 und A. Historische Einleitungen, Übersichten, Tabellen und Biographien. Der Frauenarzt 34 (1992) 561–564.

Tausk, M.: In Kracht, J., A. von zur Mühlen, P. Scriba (eds.): Endocrinology Guide. Dt. Ges. f. Endokrinologie (1976).

Welbourn, R. B.: The Pituitary, in The History of Endocrine Surgery. Praeger, New York, Westport, London (1990) 89–139.

Original-Literatur

Abraham, G. E., W. D. Odell, R. S. Swerdloff, K. Hopper: Simultaneous radioimmunoassay of Plasma FSH, LH, Progesterone, 17-Hydroxyprogesterone, and Estradiol-17β during the menstrual cycle. J. Clin. Endocr. 34 (1972) 312–318.

Acher, R., J. Chauvet: La structure de la vasopressine de boeuf. Biochem. Biophys. Acta 12 (1953) 487–488.

Acher, R., J. Chauvet, G. Olivry: Sur l'existence eventuelle d'une hormone unique neurohypophysaire. Biochim. Biophys. Acta 22 (1956) 421.

Acher, R.: Chemistry of the neurohypophysial hormone: an example of molecular evolution. In Greep, R. O., E. B. Astwood: Handbook of Physiology. Endocrinology Vol. IV, Part I (1974) 119–130.

Adler, L.: Metamorphosestudien an Batrachierlarven. Z. ges. exp. Med. 3 (1914) 39–41.

Adler, L.: Metamorphosisstudien an Batrachierlarven. A. Exstirpation der Hypophyse. Arch. Entwicklungsmech. Organ 39 (1914) 21–45.

Albert, A.: Procedure for routine clinical gonadotropin determination in human urine. Mayo Clinic Proc. 30 (1955) 552–556.

Albert, A., R. Borth, E. Diczfalusy, J. A. Loraine, B. Lunenfeld, J. W. McArthur, E. Rosemberg: Collaborative assays of two urinary preparations of human pituitary gonadotropin. J. Clin. Endocrinol. 18 (1958) 1117–1123.

Albert, A. (ed.): Human pituitary gonadotropins. Charles C. Thomas, Springfield, Illinois (1961).

Albert, A.: Large-scale separation of follicle stimulating and luteinizing hormones from male urine. Mayo Clinic Proc. 40 (1965) 312–326.

Albert, A.: The Kaolin-Aceton method for processing urine for the routine clinical assay of human pituitary gonadotrophin. Acta endocr. 52, Suppl. 106 (1966) 1–64.

Alexandridis, D. M., M. Apostolakis, K. D. Voigt: Comparative studies on methods of assay for a routine clinical gonadotropin determination in human urine. Acta endocr. 29 (1958) 537–549.

Allen, B. M.: The result of exstirpation of the anterior lobe of the hypophysis and of the thyroid of Rana Pipiens larvae. Science 44 (1916) 755–757.

Allen, B. M.: The relation of the pituitary and the thyroid glands of Bufo and Rana to iodine and metamorphosis. Biol. Bull. 36 (1919) 405–417.

Allen, B. M.: Experiments in the transplantation of the hypophysis of adult Rana pipiens to tadpoles. Science 52 (1920) 274–276.

Anderson, E. M., J. B. Collip: Thyrotropic hormone of the anterior pituitary. Proc. Soc. Exptl. Biol. Med. 30 (1923) 680–683.

Apostolakis, M.: Detection and Estimation of Pituitary Gonadotrophins in Human Plasma. J. Endocrin. 19 (1960) 377–388.

Apostolakis, M., J. A. Loraine: Renal clearance of pituitary gonadotrophins in postmenopausal women. J. cin. Endocrinol. 20 (1960) 1437–1440.

Apostolakis, M., H. Nowakowski, K. D. Voigt: Absorption and excretion of parenterally administered human pituitary gonadotropin. J. clin. Endocrinol. Metabol. 21 (1961) 575–578.

Apostolakis, M., G. Bettendorf, K. D. Voigt: Klinisch-experimentelle Studien mit menschlichem hypophysärem Gonadotropin. Acta. endocr. 41 (1962) 14–30.

Aschheim, S.: Über die Funktion des Ovarium. Zschr. Geb. Gynäk. 90 (1926) 387–392.

Aschheim, S., B. Zondek: Die Schwangerschaftsdiagnose aus dem Harn durch Nachweis des Hypophysenvorderlappenhormons. Klin. Wochenschr. 7 (1928) 1404–1411.

Aschner, B.: Demonstration von Hunden nach Exstirpation der Hypophyse. Wien klin. Wchschr. 22 (1909) 1730–1732.

Aschner, B.: Über die Beziehung zwischen Hypophyse und Genitale. Arch. Gynäk. 97 (1912) 200–228.

Aschner, B.: Über die Funktion der Hypophyse. Pflügers Arch. ges. Physiol. 146 (1912) 1–146.

Aschner, B.: Zur Physiologie des Zwischenhirns. Wien. Klin. Wschr. 25 (1912) 1042–1043.

Ascoli, G., T. Legnani: Die Folgen der Exstirpation der Hypophyse. Münch. Med. Wchschr. 59 (1912) 518–521.

Astwood, E. B.: The regulation of corpus luteum function by hypophysial luteotropin. Endocrinology 28 (1941) 309–320.

Babinski, J.: Tumeur du corps pituitaire sans acromégalie et avec arrêt de développement des organes génitaux. Rev. Neurol. Paris 8 (1900) 531–533.

Bahl, O. P.: Human chorionic gonadotropin. I Purification and physico-chemical properties. J. biol. Chem. 244 (1969) 567.

Bahl, O. P.: Human chorionic gonadotropin. II Nature of the carbohydrate units. J. biol. Chem. 244 (1969) 575.

Bahl, O. P., R. B. Carlson, R. Bellisario, N. Swaminthan: Human chorionic gonadotrophin: amino acid sequence of the α and β subunits. Biochem. biophys. Res. Commun. 48 (1972) 416–422.

Bahl, O. P.: The chemistry and biology of human chorionic gonadotropin and its subunits. In Greep, R. O., M. A. Koblinsky (eds.): Frontiers in Reproduction and Fertility Control. The MTP Press, Cambridge, Mass and London, England (1977) 11–24.

Bahn, R. C., N. Lorenz, A. W. Bennet, A. Albert: Gonadotropins of the pituitary gland and the urine of the adult human female. Endocrinology 52 (1953) 135–139.

Bangham, R., P. M. Woodward: The second international Standard for serum gonadotrophin. Bull. Wld. Hlth. Org. 35 (1966) 761–773.

Bargmann, W.: Über die neurosekretorische Verknüpfung von Hypothalamus und Neurohypophyse. Z. Zellforsch. 34 (1949) 610–634.

Bargmann, W.: Über die neurosekretorische Verknüpfung von Hypothalamus und Hypophyse. Anat. Nachr. 1 (1950) 77–78.

Bargmann, W.: Zwischenhirn und Hypophyse. Arch. Gyn. 183 (1953) 14–34.

Barker, S. A., C. J. Gray, J. F. Kennedy, W. R. Butt: Evaluation of human follicle-stimulating hormone preparations. J. Endocr. 45 (1969) 777–888.

Beck, J. C., E. E. McGarry, I. Dyrenfurth, E. H. Venning: Metabolic effects of human and monkey growth hormone in man. Science 125 (1957) 184–185.

Becker, A., A. Albert: Urinary excretion of follicle-stimulating and luteinizing hormones. J. Clin. Endocrin. Metabol. 25 (1965) 962–974.

Belchetz, P., T. M. Plant, Y. Nakai, E. J. Keogh, E. Knobil: Hypophysial responses to continuous and intermittend delivery of hypothalamic gonadotropin releasing hormone. Science 202 (1978) 631–633.

Benda, C.: Beiträge zur normalen und pathologischen Histologie der menschlichen Hypophysis cerebri. Berl. Klin. Wschr. 37 (1900) 1205–1210.

Bern, H. A., C. S. Nicoll: The comparative endocrinology of prolactin. Rec. Progr. Horm. Res. 24 (1968) 681–720.

Berthold, A. A.: Transplantation der Hoden. Arch. Anat. Physiol. u. wiss. Medizin, Berlin 2 (1849) 42–46.

Bettendorf, G., M. Apostolakis, K. D. Voigt: Darstellung von Gonadotropin aus menschlichen Hypophysen. Acta endocrinol. 41 (1962) 1–13.

Bettendorf, G., M. Breckwoldt, K. Knoerr, H. E. Stegner: Gravidität nach Hypophysektomie und Behandlung mit hypophysärem Humangonadotropin. Dtsch. Med. Wchschr. 41 (1964) 1952–1957.

Bettendorf, G.: Gonadotrophins in Human Pituitaries. Acta endocrinol. Suppl. 101 (1965) 7–8.

Bettendorf, G., D. Ahrens, K. Groot, J. H. Napp: Akutes Meigs Syndrom und Gravidität nach Ovulationsauslösung mit hypophysärem Humangonadotropin. Geburtsh. u. Frauenheilk. 25 (1965) 673–694.

Bettendorf, G., M. Breckwoldt, Ch. Neale: FSH and LH dose response relationship in ovulation induction with human gonadotropins. In Rosemberg, E. (ed.): Gonadotropins. Geron-X, Los Altos, Calif. (1968) 453–458.

Bettendorf, G., M. Breckwoldt, P. J. Czygan, A. Fock, T. Kumaska: Fractionation of human pituitary gonadotropins (extraction, gelfiltration and electrofocusing). In Rosemberg, E. (ed.): Gonadotropins. Geron-X, Los-Altos, Calif. (1968) 13–24

Bettendorf, G., M. Breckwoldt, Ch. Neale: In Louwrens: Menschliche Gonadotropine (1970). Acta endocrinol., Suppl. 64 (1968) 148.

Bettendorf, G., V. Insler: Clinical Application of Human Gonadotropins, Proceedings of a workshop Conference Hamburg 1970. Georg Thieme Verlag, Stuttgart (1970).

Bettendorf, G., F. Leidenberger: Use of desialo-hCG in induction of ovulation. In Crosignani, P. G., R. Mishell: Ovulation in the human. Acad. Press, New York (1976) 289–292.

Bettendorf, G., W. Braendle, Ch. Sprotte, Ch. Weise, R. Zimmermann: Overall Results of Gonadotropin Therapy. In Insler, V., G. Bettendorf: Advances in Diagnosis and Treatment of infertility. Elsevier / North Holland (1981) 21–26.

Bettendorf, G., W. Braendle, C. Weise, W. Poels: Effect of gonadotropin treatment during inhibited pituitary function. In Insler, V., G. Bettendorf (ed.): Advances in diagnosis and treatment of infertility. Elsevier, North Holland (1981) 43–52.

Bettendorf, G., W. Braendle, Ch. Sprotte, V. Poels, V. Lichtenberg, Ch. Lindner: Pharmacologic Hypogonadotropism – an advantage for hMG-induced follicular maturation and succeeding fertilization. Horm. metabol. Res. 18 (1986) 656–657.

Bettendorf, G., Ch. Lindner: The Ovarian Hyperstimulation Syndrome. Horm. Metabol. Res. 19 (1987) 519–522.

Blaire Bell, W.: The pituitary body and the action of pituitary extract in shock, uterine atony and intestinal paresis. Brit. med. J. part. 2 (1909) 1609–1613.

Bhalla, V. K., L. E. Reichert: Gonadotropin receptors in rat testis. J. Biol. Chem. 249 (1974) 7996–8004.

Binz, F.: Besteht die Möglichkeit, die Wachstumsanregung des Uterus zur Serodiagnostik zu verwenden? Münch. med. Wchschr. 2 (1924) 899.

Birkhäuser, M.: Ovarielle Stimulation mit einem „reinen" FSH-Präparat beim Polyzystischen Ovarsyndrom. In Lehmann, F., M. Breckwoldt (Hrsg.): Gonadotropine, HMG-Behandlung in der Praxis. Bücherei des Frauenarztes 39 (1991) 31–40.

Blobel, R., H. Uhlig, G. Schumacher: Biochemical studies with human chorionic gonadotrophin (HCG). Acta endocrinol. 67 (1962) 72–76.

Blobel, R.: Über das Choriongonadotropin, Untersuchungen zur biologischen Charakterisierung verschiedener Präparationen. Karker, Basel, New York, Fortschr. Geburtsh. Gynäk. 28 (1966).

Bogdanove, E. M., N. B. Schwartz, L. E. Reichert, A. R. Midgley: Comparison of pituitary: serum LH ratios in the castrated rat by radioimmunoassay and OAAD bioassay. Endocrinol. 88 (1971) 644–652.

Bonet, Th.: Sepulchretum sive anatomica ex cadaveribus morbo donatis. L. Chouet, Genevae (1979).

Borth, R., B. Lunenfeld, H. de Watteville: Activité gonadotrope d'un extrait d'urines de femmes en menopause. Experientia 10 (1954) 266–270.

Borth, R., B. Lunenfeld, G. Riotton, H. de Watteville: Activité gonadotrope d'un extrait d'urines de femmes en menopause (2me communication) Experientia 13 (1957) 115–121.

Borth, R., B. Lunenfeld, H. de Watteville: Day-to-day variation in urinary gonadotrophin and steroid levels during the normal menstrual cycle. Fertil. Steril. 8 (1957) 233–254.

Borth, R., E. Diczfalusy, H. D. Heinrichs: Grundlagen der statistischen Auswertung biologischer Bestimmungen. Arch. Gynäk. 188 (1957) 497.

Bowers, C. Y., K. Folkers, Knudsen et al.: Hypothalamic peptide hormones, chemistry and physiology. In DeGroot, L.: Endocrinology, Vol I. Grune & Stratton, New York, San Francisco, London (1979) 65–93.

Bradbury, J. T.: The Estrous rabbit as a quantitative assay animal. Endocrinology 35 (1944) 317–324.

Bradbury, J. T.: After Office Hours – Die innere Sekretion von Ovarium und Plazenta und ihre Bedeutung für die Funktion der Milchdrüse. Privatdozent Dr. Josef Halban. Obstet. Gynecol. 6 (1985) 559–565.

Braendle, W., S. Starcevic, G. Bettendorf: Effect of an FSH preparation with low LH activity in ovarian insufficiency displaying high LH/FSH ratio. In Insler, V., G. Bettendorf (eds.): Advances in Diagnosis and Treatment of Infertility. Elseviere/North Holland, Amsterdam (1981) 33–41.

Breckwoldt, M., G. Bettendorf: Gonadotropin-Bestimmung bei der Ovarialinsuffizienz mit Hilfe von Antikörpern gegen Choriongonadotropin. Endokrinologie 50 (1966) 162–167.

Breckwoldt, M., P. J. Czygan, G. Bettendorf: Extraction of LH-preparations from human pituitaries. Acta endocrin. Suppl. 119 (1967) 128.

Breckwoldt, M., G. Bettendorf: Induction of Ovulation in the non-cycling Rhesus Monkey (Macaca Mulatta) with various gonadotropins. In Bettendorf, G., V. Insler (ed.): Clinical Application of Human Gonadotropins. G. Thieme, Stuttgart (1970) 160–162.

Breckwoldt, M., P. J. Czygan, F. Lehmann, G. Bettendorf: Synthetic LH-RH as therapeutic Agent. Acta endocrinol. 75 (1974) 209–220.

Brody, S., G. Carlström: Serologic determination of hCG in body fluids. Lancet 2 (1960) 99.

Brody, S., G. Carlström: Immuno-assay of human chorionic gonadotropin in normal and pathological pregnancy. J. Clin. Endocrinol. Metabol. 22 (1961) 564–574.

Brossmer, R., M. Dörner, U. Hilgenfeldt, F. Leidenberger, E. Trude: Purification and characterization of human chorionic gonadotropin. FEBS letters 15 (1971) 33–35.

Brossmer, R., W. E. Merz, U. Hilgenfeldt: Separation of purified human chorionic gonadotropin into single bands by isoelectro focusing and their characterization. FEBS letters 18 (1971) 112–114.

Brown, J. B., A. Klopper, J. A. Loraine: The urinary excretion of oestrogens, pregnanediol and gonadotrophins during the menstrual cycle. J. endocrinol. 17 (1958) 401–410.

Brown, J. B., S. C. McLeod, C. Macnaughtan, M. A. Smith, B. Smith: A rapid method for estimating oestrogens in urine using a semiautomatic extractor. J. endocrinol. 42 (1968) 5–15.

Brown, J. B.: In Bettendorf, G.: Zur Geschichte der Endokrinologie und Reproduktionsmedizin. Springer Verlag (1995) 67–69.

Brown, J. B.: Gonadotropins. In Insler, V., B. Lunenfeld: Infertility: Male and Female. Churchill Livingstone, Edinburgh, London, Melbourne, New York (1986) 359–396.

Brown, J. N., J. H. Evans, F. D. Adey, H. P. Taft, L. Townsend: Factors involved in the induction of fertile ovulations with human gonadotrophins. J. Obstet. Gynecol. Br. Commonw. 76 (1969) 289–307.

Brown, P. S.: Follicle stimulating and interstitial cell stimulating hormones in the urine of women with amenorrhoea. J. Endocrin. 14 (1956) 129–137.

Brown, P. S.: Human urinary gonadotrophins I. in relation to puberty. J. Endocrin. 17 (1958) 329–336.

Brown, W. E., J. T. Bradbury: A study of the physiologic action of human chorionic hormone. The production of pseudopregnancy in women by chorionic hormone. Am. J. Obstet. Gynec. 53 (1947) 749–757.

Browne, J. S. L., E. H. Venning: The effect of intramuscular injection of gonadotropic substances on the corpus luteum phase of the human menstrual cycle. Am. J. Physiol. 123 (1938) 6.

Buchholz, R.: Untersuchungen über die Ausscheidungsverhältnisse der gonadotropen Hypophysenhormone FSH und LH im menstruellen Cyclus. Z. gesamte exp. Medizin 128 (1957) 219–242.

Buchholz, R.: Quantitative Bestimmung der gonadotropen Hypophysenhormone im Zyklus. Geburts. Frhkd. 17 (1957) 707–716.

Burch, J. C., R. S. Cunningham: Effect of placental extracts on ovarian stimulating properties of anterior hypophysis. Proc. Soc. Exp. Biol. Med. 27 (1929) 331–332.

Burgos, R., M. Butcher, N. Ling, R. Guillemin: Structure moleculair du facteur hypothylamique (LRF) d'origine ovine controlant la secretion de l'hormone gonadotrope hypophysaire luteinisation. C. R. Acid. Sci. 273 (1971) 1611–1613.

Büttner, W.: Die Wirkung des Follikelhormons und der gonadotropen Hormone bei der Frau in anatomischer und funktioneller Betrachtung. (Habilitationsschrift Bonn). Arch. Gynäk. 163 (1937) 487–551.

Butt, W. R., A. C. Crooke, F. J. Cunningham: Studies on human urinary and pituitary gonadotrophins. Biochem. J. 81 (1961) 596–605.

Buvat, J., J. L. Dehaene, M. Buvat-Herbaut, P. Verbecq, G. Marcolin, O. Renouard: Purified FSH in PCOs. Slow administration is safer and more effective. Fertil. Steril. 52 (1989) 553–558.

Buxton, C. L., W. Herrmann: Induction of ovulation in the humans with human gonadotropins. Am. J. Obstet. Gynec. 81 (1961) 584.

Campbell, A. D., J. B. Collip: On the clinical use of the ovary-stimulating hormone of the placenta. Canad. Med. Ass. J. 22 (1930) 219–220.

Canfield, R. E., F. J. Morgan, S. Kammermann, J. J. Bell, G. M. Agusto: Studies of human chorionic gonadotropin. Rec. Progr. Horm. Res. 27 (1971) 121.

Caspi, E., J. Ronen, P. Schreyer, M. D. Goldberg: The outcome of pregnancy after gonadotrophin therapy. Br. J. Obstet. Gynecol. 83 (1976) 967.

Caton, R., F. T. Paul: Notes on a case of acromegaly treated by operation. Br. Med. J. 2 (1893) 1421–1423.

Catt, K. J., M. L. Dufau, T. Tsuruhara: Radioligand receptor assay of luteinzing hormone and chorionic gonadotropins. J. Clin. Endocr. Metab. 34 (1972) 123–132.

Chappel, S., C. Kelton, N. Nugent: Expression of human gonadotropins by recombinant DNA methods. In Genazzani, A. R.: Petraglia, Fed. Proc. 3. World Congr. Gyn. Endocrinol. The Parhenon Publ. Group (1992) 179–184.

Chretien, M.: Lipotropins. In Berson, S., R. Yalow: Peptide Hormones. Vol. 2A. Amsterdam, North Holland (1973) 617.

Claesson, L., B. Hoberg, T. Rosenberg, A. Westman: Cristalline human chorionic gonadotropin and its biological action. Acta endocrinol. 1 (1948) 1.

Claman, P., M. M. Seibel: Purified Human Follicle-Stimulating Hormone for Ovulation Induction. Seminars in Reproductive Endocrinology 4 (1986) 277–284.

Clauberg, C.: Die einmalige Transfusion einer größeren Menge Schwangerenblutes als Ersatztherapie bei pathologischen Blutungen der Uterusschleimhaut infolge Follikelpersistenz im Ovar. Zbl. Gynäk. 57 (1933) 47–48.

Clauberg, C.: Die weiblichen Sexualhormone in ihren Beziehungen zum Genitalzyklus und zum Hypophysenvorderlappen. J. Springer, Berlin (1933).

Cochius, J. L., K. Mack, R. J. Burns: Creutzfeld-Jakob disease in a recipient human pituitary derived gonadotrophin. Aust. N. Z. J. Med. 20 (1990) 592.

Cole, H. H., G. H. Hart: The potency of blood serum of mares in progressive stages of pregnancy in effecting the sexual maturity of the immature rat. Am. J. Physiol. 93 (1930) 57–68.

Collip, J. B.: The ovarian-stimulating hormone of the placenta. Peliminary paper. Can. Med. Ass. J. 22 (1930) 219–220.

Corner, G. W.: The hormonal control of lactation I. Non-effect of the corpus luteum. II. Positive action of extracts of the hypophysis. Am. J. Physiol. 95 (1930) 43–55.

Corral, J., J. Calderon, J. W. Goldzieher: Induction of Ovulation and Term Pregnancy in a Hypohysectomized Woman. Obstetrics and Gynecology 39 (1972) 397–400.

Cotonnec, le J. Y., H. C. Porchet, V. Beltrami, A. Khan, S. Toon, M. R. Rowland: Clinical pharmacology of recombinant human follicle-stimulating hormone (FSH) I. Comparative pharmacokinetics with urinary human FSH. Fertil. Steril. 61, 669–678 – II. Single doses and steady state pharmacokinetics. Fertil. Steril. 61 (1994) 679–695.

Courrier, R., R. Guillemin, M. Jutisz, E. Sakiz, P. Aschheim: Presence dans un extrait d'hypothalamus d'une substance qui stimule la secretion de l'hormone antehypophysaire de luteinisation. C. R. Acad. Sci. 253 (1961) 922–927.

Crowe, S. J., H. Cushing, J. Homans: Effects of hypophyseal transplantation following total hypophysectomy in the canine. Johns Hopkins Univ. Quart J. Exptl. Physiol. 2 (1909) 389–400.

Crowe, S. J., H. Cushing, J. Homans: Experimental hypophysectomy. The Johns Hopkins Hosp. Bull. 21 (1910) 127–169.

Crooke, A. C., W. R. Butt, R. F. Palmer, R. Morris, R. L. Edwards, C. J. Anson: Clinical trial of human gonadotrophins I – The effect of pituitary and urinary FSH and hCG on patients with idiopathic secondary amenorrhoea. J. Ob. Gyn. Brit. Comwth. LXX (1963) 604–631.

Crooke, A. C., W. R. Butt, S. P. Carrington, R. Morris, R. F. Palmer, R. L. Edwards: Pregnancy im women with secondary amenorrhoea treated with human gonadotrophins. Lancet (1964) 184–188.

Crooke, A. C., W. R. Butt, P. V. Betrand: Treatment of idiopathic secondary amenorrhoea with single injections of FSH and hCG. Lancet (1966) 514–516.

Crooke, A. C., W. R. Butt, P. V. Bertrand, R. Morris: Treatment of infertility and secondary amenorrhoea with FSH and hCG. Lancet (1967) 636–637.

Crooke, A. C., G. Eleftheriadis, P. V. Bertrand: Induction of Ovulation with Human Gonadotrophins: Factor Affecting Ovulation, Pregnancy and Complications. Hormones 1 (1970) 46–72.

Crooke, A. C., U. D. Saturia, P. V. Bertrand: Comparison of daily with twice-weekly injections of FSH for treatment of failure of ovulation. Am. J. Obst. Gyn. 111 (1971) 405 – 412.

Cseh, G., E. Barat, L. Graf: Studies on the primary structure of human β-lipotropin hormone. FEBS Lett. 21 (1972) 344 – 345.

Currie, A. R., J. B. Dekanski: Gonadotrophins and Prolactin in human pituitary glands. Acta endocrin. 36 (1961) 185 – 196.

Cushing, H. W.: The functions of the pituitary body. Am. J. Med. Sci. 139 (1910) 473 – 484.

Cushing, H. W.: The hypophysis cerebri. Clinical aspects of hyperpituitarism and of hypopituitarism. J. Am. Med. Ass. 53 (1909) 249 – 255.

Cushing, H. W.: The pituitary body and its disorders. J. P. Lippincott, Philadelphia and London (1912).

Cushing, H. W.: Intracranial Tumours. Springfield, Illinois (1932).

Czygan, P. J.: Regulationsprinzipien der weiblichen Keimdrüsenfunktion. Fortschr. Geb. Gynäk. 52 (1974) 121 – 198.

Dale, H. H.: On some physiological actions of ergot. J. Physiol. London 34 (1906) 165 – 206.

Dale, H. H.: The action of extracts of the pituitary body. Biochem. J. 4 (1909) 427 – 447.

Damme, van M. P., D. M. Robertson, R. Marana, Ritzén, E. Diczfalusy: A sensitive and specific in vitro bioassay method for the measurement of follicle-stimulating hormone activity. Acta endocrinol. 91 (1979) 224 – 237.

Daume, E., G. Dörner: Klinische Resultate der Amenorrhöbehandlung mit der Kombination Choriongonadotropin und hypophysäres FSH. III Weltkongr. Int. Fed. Gyn. Geburtsh., Wien Bd. II (1961) 292.

Davies, A. G.: Eunuchoid treated with gonadotrophins. Proc. roy. Soc. Med. 58 (1964) 580.

Davis, M. E., A. K. Koff: The experimental production of ovulation in the human subject. Am. J. Obstet. Gynec. 36 (1938) 183 – 199.

Davis, M. E., A. A. Hellbaum: Observations on the experimental use of gonadotropic extracts in the human female. J. clin. Endocr. 4 (1944) 400.

De la Llosa, C. Courte, M. Jutisz: On the mechanism of reversible inactivation of luteinizing hormone by urea. Biochem. Biophys. Res. Commun. 226 (1967) 411 – 416.

De la Llosa, M. Jutisz: Reversible dissociation with subunits and biological activity of ovine luteinizing hormone. Biochim. Biophys. Acta 181 (1969) 426 – 436.

Del Pozo, E., R. Brun, L. Varga, H. Friesen: The inhibition of prolactin secretion in man by CB 154 (2. Bromo-alpha-ergocryptine). J. Clin. Endocr. Metab. 35 (1972) 768 – 770.

Del Pozo, E., H. G. Friesen, P. Burmeister: Endocrine profile of a specific prolactin inhibitor: Br. ergocryptine (CB 154). Schweiz. Med. Wschr. 103 (1973) 847 – 850.

Devroey, P., A. van Steirtegem, B. Mannaerts, K. Coeling Bennink: Succesful in vitro fertilization and embryo transfer after treatment with recombinant human FSH. Lancet 339 (1992) 1170 – 1171.

Devroey, P., B. Mannaerts, J. Smitz, H. Coelingh Bennink, A. van Steirteghem: First established pregnancy and birth after ovarian stimulation with recombinant human follicle stimulating hormone (Org 32489). Human Reprod. 8 (1993) 863 – 865.

Dietel, F. G.: Das gonadotrope Hormon des Hypophysenvorderlappens. Ber. ges. Gynäk. Geburtsh. 27 (1934) 369 – 448.

Diczfalusy, E.: Chorionic gonadotrophin and estrogens in the human placenta. Acta Endocrinol. Suppl. 12 (1953) 1 – 175.

Diczfalusy, E., P. Troen: Endocrine functions of the human placenta. Vitam. and Horm. 19 (1961) 230.

Diczfalusy, E., E. Johannison, K. G. Tillinger, G. Bettendorf: Comparison of the clinical and steroid metabolic effect of human pituitary and urinary gonadotropins in amenorrhoeic women. Acta endocrinol. Suppl. 90 (1964) 35–56.

Dierschke, D. J., A. N. Bhattacharya, L. E. Atkinson, E. Knobil: Circhoral oscillations of plasma LH levels in the ovariectomized Rhesus monkey. Endocrinol. 87 (1970) 850–853.

Dodd, J. M.: Ovarian Control in Cyclostomes and Elasmobranchs. Am. Zoologist 12 (1972) 325 –339.

Dörner, G., E. Daume: Über die Wirkung der Hormonkombination follikelstimulierendes Hormon und Choriongonadotropin auf die Ovarien amenorrhoischer Frauen. Klin. Wschr. 39 (1961) 1260.

Dörner, G., W. Hohlweg, E. Daume: Über die synergistische Wirkung von Gonadotropin-kombinationen auf das Ovar. III. Weltkongr. Int. Fed. Gynäk. Geburtsh. Wien, Berichte Bd. II (1961) 290.

Dörner, G., F. Döcke: Geschlechtsspezifische Reaktion des Hypothalamus-Hypophysenvor-derlappensystems der Ratte nach einmaliger Östrogenapplikation. Z. Gynäkol. 86 (1964) 1321–1323.

Donaldson, E. M., F. Yamazaki, H. M. Dye, W. W. Philleo: Preparation of Gonadotropin from Salmon (Oncorhynchus tshawytscha) pituitary glands. Gen. comp. Endocrinol. 18 (1972) 469–480.

Donini, P., M. Montezemolo: Gonadotropina preipofisaria e gonadotropina preipofiso-simi-le umana. Rass. Clin. Ter. Sc. Aff. 48 (1949) 143–152.

Donini, P., D. Puzzuoli, R. Montezemulo: Purification of gonadotrophin from menopausal urine. Acta endocr. 45 (1964) 321–328.

Donini, P., D. Puzzuoli, I. D'Alessio: Purification of gonadotrophin from menopausal urine by gel filtration on sephadex. Acta endocr. 45 (1964) 329–334.

Donini, P., D. Puzzuoli, I. D'Alessio, B. Lunenfeld, A. Eshkol, A.F. Parlow: Purification and separation of FSH and LH from human Menopausalgonadotropin. II. Preparation of biological apparently pure FSH by selective binding of the LH with an anti-hCG serum and subsequently chromatography. Acta endocr. 52 (1966) 186–198.

Donini, P., D. Puzzuoli, I. D'Alessio, S. Donini: Human Follicle-stimulating Hormone. Pu-rification and some biological properties. Pharmacology of hormonal Polypeptides and Proteins. Plenum Press (1968) 229–238.

Donini, P., D. Puzzouli, L. D'Alessio, S. Donini: A new approach to the biological determi-nation of the luteinizing hormone. Acta endocrin. 58 (1968) 463.

Dufau, M. L., R. Pock, A. Neubauer, K. J. Catt: In vitro bioassay of LH in human serum: The rat interstitial cell testerone (RICT) assay. J. Endocrinol. Metab. 42 (1976) 969–985.

Dumble, L. D., R. D. Klein: Creutzfeld-Jakob disease legacy for Australian women treated with human pituitary gonadotropins. Lancet 340 (1992) 848–850.

Dyke, van H. B., H. C. Coffin: Proposed names for the follicle stimulating hormone and interstitial-cell stimulating hormone of the anterior lobe of the pituitary body. Science 93 (1941) 61–63.

Ehrhardt, K., B. T. Mayes: Beitrag zum Hormongehalt des menschlichen und tierischen Hypophysenvorderlappen. Zbl. Gynäk. 44 (1930) 2949–2952.

Eiselsberg, A. von, L. von Frankl-Hochwart: Über operative Behandlung der Hypophysistu-moren. Wien Klin. Wschr. 20 (1907) 1341.

Eiselsberg, A. von: Zur Operation der Hypophysisgeschwülste. Arch. Klin. Chir. 100 (1912) 13–37.

Ellis, S.: Bioassay of luteinizing hormon. Endocrinology 68 (1961) 334–340.

Elrick, H., V. Yearwood-Drayton, Y. Arai, H. G. Morris: Hormonal content of pituitaries from embalmed bodies. J. Clin. Endocrin. Metab. 24 (1964) 910–914.

Engel, T., R. Jewelewicz, I. Dyrenfurth, L. Spiroff, R. L. van de Wiele: Ovarian hyperstimulation syndrome. Am. J. Obstet. Gynecol. 112 (1972) 1052–1060.

Eppinger, H., W. Falta, C. Rudinger: Über die Wechselwirkung der Drüsen mit innerer Sekretion. Z. f. klin. Med. 66 (1908) 1–52.

Erdheim, J.: Zur normalen und pathologischen Histologie der Glandula thyroidea, Parathyroidea und Hypophysis. Beitr. Pathol. Anat. 33 (1903) 158–236.

Erdheim, J.: Sitzungsbericht Kais. Akad. Wiss. Mathem. Naturwiss. Kl. Wien 113 (1904) 537.

Erdheim, J.: Nanosomia pituitaria. Zieglers Beitr. 62 (1916) 302–377.

Eshkol, A., B. Lunenfeld: Purification and separation of FSH and LH from human menopausal gonadotrophin (hMG). Acta endocrinol. 54 (1967) 919–931.

Evans, H. M., J. A. Long: The effect of the anterior lobe administered intraperitoncally upon the growth, maturity and the oestrus cycle of the rat. Anat. Rec. 21 (1921) 62–63.

Evans, H. M., J. A. Long: Characteristic effects upon growth, oestrus and ovulation induced by the intraperitoneal administration of fresh anterior hypophyseal substance. Proc. Nat. Acid. Sci. 8 (1922) 38–39.

Evans, H. M., M. E. Simpson: Hyperplasia of the mammary apparatus of adult virgin females induced by anterior hypophyseal hormones. Proc. Soc. Exptl. Biol. Med. 26 (1929) 598.

Evans, H. M., M. E. Simpson: Hormones of the anterior hypophysis. Am. J. Physiol. 98 (1931) 511–546.

Evans, H. M., K. Meyer, M. E. Simpson: The growth and gonad-stimulating hormones of the anterior hypophysis. Mem. Univ. Calif. 2 (1933) 67–229.

Evans, H. M.: Clinical manifestations of dysfunction of the anterior pituitary. In Glandular Physiology and Therapy, Chicago, Am. Med. Assoc. 7 (1935).

Evans, H. M., M. E. Simpson, R. I. Pencharz: „Deficiency" changes in the testicular Leydig cells after hypophysectomy. Proc. 51. Session of Am. Assn. of Anatomists. Anat. Rec., Suppl. 61 (1935) 44.

Evans, H. M., K. Korpi, M. E. Simpson, R. I. Pencharz, D. H. Wonder: On the separation of the interstitial cell-stimulating, luteinizing and follicle-stimulating fractions in the anterior pituitary gonadotropic complex. Univ. Calif. Publs. Anat. 1 (1936) 255–274.

Evans, H. M., K. Korpi, R. I. Pencharz, D. H. Wonder: On the separation of the interstitial cell-stimulating, luteinizing, and follicle-stimulating fractions in the anterior pituitary gonadotropic complex. Univ. California Publ. Anat. 1 (1936) 255–273.

Evans, H. M., M. E. Simpson, R. I. Pencharz: An anterior pituitary gonadotropic fraction (ICSH) specifically stimulating the interstitial tissue of testis and ovary. Cold Spring Harbor Symp. Quant. Biol. 5 (1937) 229–240.

Evans, H. M., M. E. Simpson, R. I. Pencharz: Biological studies of the gonadotropic principles in sheep pituitary substance. Endocrinol. 25 (1939) 529–546.

Evans, H. M., M. E. Simpson, W. R. Lyons: Influence of lactogenic preparations on production of traumatic placentoma in rat. Proc. Soc. Exptl. Biol. Med. 46 (1941) 586–590.

Evans, H. M., M. E. Simpson, W. R. Lyons, K. Turpeinen: Anterior pituitary hormones which favor production of traumatic uterine placentoma. Endocrinology 28 (1941) 933–945.

Evans, H. M., M. E. Simpson, W. Marx, E. Kibrick: Bioassay of the pituitary growth hormone. Width of the proximal epiphyseal cartilage of the tibia in hypophysectomized rats. Endocrinology 32 (1943) 13–16.

Faiman, C., J. S. D. Winter: Sex differences in gonadotrophin concentrations in infancy. Nature 232 (1971) 130–131.

Farini, F.: Diabete insipido éd opoterapia. Gazz. Osped. Clin. 34 (1913) 1135–1139.

Fellner, O. O.: Experimentelle Untersuchungen über die Wirkung von Gewebsextrakten aus der Plazenta und den weiblichen Sexualorganen auf das Genitale. Arch. Gyn. 100 (1913) 641–719.

Fevold, H. L., F. L. Hisaw, S. L. Leonard: The gonad stimulating and the luteinizing hormones of the anterior lobe of the hypophysis. Am. J. Physiol. 97 (1931) 291–301.

Fevold, H. L., F. L. Hisaw: Interactions of gonad stimulating hormone in ovarian development. Am. J. Physiol. 109 (1934) 655–665.

Fevold, H. L.: The gonadotrophic hormones. Cold Spring Harbor Symposium. Quant. Biol. 5 (1937) 93–103.

Figuera-Cases, P.: Reaccion ovarica monstrosa a las gonadotropinas a proposito de un caso fatal. Ann. Cirurg. 23 (1958) 116.

Floyd, W. S., L. Cohn: Gonadotropin producing hepatoma. Obst. Gynecol. 41 (1972) 665–668.

Flückiger, E., P. M. Lutterbeck, H. R. Wagner, E. Billeter: Antagonism of 2. Bromo-alpha-ergocryptine-methansulfonate (CB 154) to certain endocrine actions of centraly active drugs. Experientia 28 (1972) 924–926.

Fluhmann, C. F.: Anterior pituitary hormone in the blood of women with ovarian deficiency. JAMA 93 (1929) 672–674.

Foges, A., R. Hofstätter: Über Pituitrinwirkung bei post-partum Blutungen. Zbl. Gynäkol. 34 (1910) 1500–1504.

Franchimont, P.: Le dosage des hormones hypophysaires somatotropes et gonadique et son application clinique. Arscia, Bruxelles, Maloine, Paris (1967).

Franchimont, P., J. L. Pasteels: Sécrétion indépendante des hormones gonadotropes et de leurs sous-unités. C. r. Sci. Paris 275 (1972) 1799–1802.

Franchimont, P., U. Gaspard, A. Reuter, G. Heynen: Polymorphism of Protein and Polypeptide Hormones. Clin. Endocrinol. 1 (1972) 315–336.

Frankl-Hochwart, von L., A. Fröhlich: Zur Kenntnis der Wirkung des Hypophysins auf das sympathische und autonome Nervensystem. Arch. exptl. Pathol. Pharmakol. 63 (1909) 347–356.

Friedman, M. H.: Mechanism of ovulation in the rabbit. II Ovulation produced by the injection of urine from pregnant women. Am. J. Ophysiol. 90 (1929) 617–622.

Friesen, M. H., H. Guyda, J. Hardy: Biosynthesis of human growth hormone and prolactin. J. Cli. Endocrinol. Metab. 31 (1970) 611–624.

Friesen, H. G., P. Hwang, H. Guyda, G. Tollis, J. Tyson, R. Myers: A radioimmunoassay for human prolactin. In Boyns, A. R., K. Griffiths (ed.): Forth Tenvous Workshop, Prolactinand Carcinogenesis. Cardiff, Wales (1972) 64–80.

Friesen, H. G., P. Hwang: The purification of human and monkey prolactin. In Josimovich, J. B., M. Reynolds, E. Cobo (ed.): Lactogenic Hormones, Fetal nutrition and Lactation. Wiley, New York (1974) 1–18.

Fritzsche, Ch. F., Th. A. E. Klebs: Ein Beitrag zur Pathologie des Riesenwuchses. Leipzig (1884).

Fröhlich, A.: Ein Fall von Tumor der Hypophysis cerebri ohne Akromegalic. Wien. Klin. Rundschau 15 (1901) 883–886 u. 906–908.

Fukushima, M., V. C. Stevens, C. L. Gantt, N. Vorys: Urinary FSH and LH excretion during the normal menstrual cycle. J. Clin. Endocrinol. 24 (1964) 205–213.

Gaddum, J. H.: Some properties of the separated active principles of the pituitary (posterior lobe). J. Physiol., London 65 (1928) 434–440.

Gadner, H., B. Weber, H. Riehm: Adrenocortical carcinoma with ectopic LH Production. Z. Kinderheilk. 118 (1974) 63–70.

Gay, V. L., A. R. Midgley, G. D. Niswender: Patterns of gonadotrophin secretion – associated with ovulation. Federation Proc. 29 (1970) 1880–1887.

Gay, V. L., N. A. Sheth: Evidence for a periodic release of LH in castrated male and female rats. Endocrinology 90 (1972) 158–162.

Gemzell, C., E. Diczfalusy, K. G. Tillinger: Clinical effect of human pituitary follicle-stimulating hormone (FSH). J. Clin. Endocrinol. Metab. 18 (1958) 1333–1348.

Gemzell, C., E. Diczfalusy, K. G. Tillinger: Human Pituitary Follicle-Stimulating Hormone. I. Clinical Effect of a partially purified preparation. Ciba Found. Coll. on Endocrinology „Human Pituitary Hormones“ G.E.W. Wolstenholme u. Connor, OConnor, C. M., J. A. Churchill, London 13 (1960) 191–208.

Gemzell, C.: Induction of ovulation with human pituitary gonadotrophins. Fertil. Steril. 13 (1962) 153.

Gemzell, C.: Induction of ovulation with human gonadotropins. II Int. Congr. Endocrinology London. Excerpta Med. Found. Int. Congr. Ser. 83 (1964).

Gemzell, C., B. Kjessler: Treatment of infertility after partial hypophysectomy with human pituitary gonadotropins. Lancet 1 (1964) 644–646.

Gemzell, C., P. Roos: Pregnancies following treatment with human gonadotropins. With special reference to the problem of multiple birth. Am. J. Obstet. Gynecol. 94 (1966) 490–496.

Gemzell, C.: Induction of Ovulation in patients following removal of a pituitary adenoma. Am. J. Obstet. Gyn. 117 (1973) 955–961.

Gemzell, C., C. F. Wang: Outcome of pregnancy in women with pituitary adenoma. Fertil. Steril. 31 (1979) 363–372.

Germond, M., S. Dessole, A. Senn, E. Loumaye, C. Howles, V. Beltrami: Successful in vitro fertilization and embryo transfer after treatment with recombinant human FSH. Lancet 339 (1992) 1170.

Gey, G. O., G. E. S. Jones, L. M. Hellman: The production of a gonadotrophic substance (prolan) by placental cells in tissue culture. Science 88 (1938) 306.

Glass, R. H., G. van Wagenen: Immunological test for chorionic gonadotropin in serum of the pregnant monkey (Macaca mulatta). Proc. Soc. Exp. Biol. Med. 134 (1970) 467–468.

Glinski, L. K.: Anatomische Veränderungen der Hypophyse. Dtsch. Med. Wochenschr. 39 (1913) 473.

Goebelsmann, U., A. R. Midgley, R. Jaffe: Regulation of human gonadotropins: VII. Daily individual urinary estrogens, pregnanediol and serum luteinizing and follicle stimulating hormones during the menstrual cacle. J. Clin. Endocr. 29 (1969) 1222–1230.

Goecke, H.: Die klinischen Erscheinungen bei Hyperplasia glandularis cystica. Zbl. Gynäk. 59 (1935) 788.

Gorbman, A.: Ultrafiltration of urine for collection and biological assay of extracted hypophyseal hormones. Endocrinology 37 (1945) 177–181.

Got, R.: Récent Acquisitions sur la Gonadotropine choriale humaine. Path. Biol. 8 (1960) 1583–1592.

Got, R., R. Bourrillon: Nouvelles donnés physiques sur la gonadotropine choriale humaine. Biochim. Biophys. Acta 39 (1960) 241.

Gottfried, S.: Hypophysenextrakt als Wehenmittel. Zbl. Gynäkol. 35 (1911) 542–543.

Graesslin, D., Y. Yaoi, G. Bettendorf: Purification of human pituitary FSH and LH controlled by disc electrophoresis and carbohydrate analysis. In Butt, W. R., A. C. Crooke, M. Ryle (eds.): Gonadotropins and ovarian development. E & S Livingstone, Edinburgh (1970) 15–21.

Graesslin, D., H. C. Weise, P. J. Czygan: Isolation and partial characterization of several different chorionic gonadotropin components. FEBS letters 20 (1972) 87–89.

Graesslin, D., H. C. Weise, W. Braendle: The microheterogeneity of human chorionic gonadotropin reflected in the β-subunits. FEBS letters 31 (1973) 214.

Green, J. D., G. W. Harris: The neurovascular link between the neurohypophysis and adenohypophysis. J. Endocrinol. 5 (1947) 136–147.

Greep, R. O.: Effect of follicle stimulating and luteinizing hormones on the testicles and accessories of normal and hypophysectomized rats. Anat. Rec. 64 (1935) 55.

Greep, R. O., H. L. Fevold, F. L. Hisaw: Effect of two hypophyseal gonadotropic hormones on the reproductive system of the male rat. An. Rec. 65 (1936) 261–272.

Greep, R. O.: Pituitary regulation of the male gonad. Cold Spring. Habor Symp. Quant. Biol. 5 (1937) 136–143.

Greep, R. O., H. L. Fevold: The spermatogenic and secretory function of the gonads of hypophysectomized adult rats treated with pituitary FSH and LH. Endocrinology 21 (1937) 611–618.

Greep, R. O., H. B. van Dyke, B. F. Chow: Use of anterior lobe of prostate gland in the assay of metakentrin. Proc. Soc. exp. Biol. Med. 46 (1941) 644–649.

Greep, R. O., H. B. van Dyke, B. F. Chow: Gonadotropins of the swine pituitary. I Various biological effects of purified thylakentrin (FSH) and pure metakentrin (ICSH). Endocrinol. 30 (1942) 635–649.

Gröschel, U., Ch. H. Li: On the carbohydrate moiety of ovine and human pituitary gonadotropins. Biochim. Biophs. Acta 37 (1960) 375–376.

Groot-Wassink, K.: Vergleichende Untersuchungen über Ovulationsauslösung beim Menschen durch kombinierte Verabreichung von hCG und tierischem bzw. menschlichen FSH. Zbl. Gynäkol. 89 (1967) 1240–1248.

Grüter, F.: Contribution a l'etude fu fonctionement du lobe anterieur de l'hypophyse. Compt. Rend. Soc. Biol. 96 (1928) 1215–1217.

Grüter, F., P. Stricker: Über die Wirkung eines Hypophysenvorderlappenhormons auf die Auslösung der Milchsekretion. Klin. Wchschr. 8 (1929) 3222–2323.

Gull, W. W.: On a cretinoid state supervening in adult life in women. Trans. Clin. Soc. London 7 (1874) 180–185.

Hack, M., M. Brish, D. M. Serr, V. Insler, B. Lunenfeld: Outcome of pregnancy after induced ovulation. JAMA 211 (1970) 791.

Hackeloer, B. J., S. Nitschke, E. Daume, G. Sturm, R. Buchholz: Ultraschalldarstellung von Ovarveränderungen bei Gonadotropinstimulierung. Geburtsh. Frauenheilk. 37 (1977) 185–190.

Hackeloer, B. J., R. Dörfler, S. Nitschke, R. Buchholz: Ultraschalldarstellung des Follikelwachstums und Basaltemperaturmessung – Vergleich zweier Methoden zur Ovulationsbestimmung. Ultraschall 1 (1980) 133–139.

Hagen, C., A. S. McNeilly: Identification of human luteinizing hormone, follicle stimulating hormone, luteinizing hormone β-subunit and gonadotrophin α-subunit in foetal and adult pituitary glands. J. Endocr. 67 (1975) 49–57.

Hagen, C., A. S. McNeilly: The gonadotrophins and their subunits in foetal pituitary glands and circulation. J. Steroid. Biochem. 8 (1977) 537–544.

Haighton, J.: An experimental inquiry concerning animal impragnation. Phil. Trans. R. Soc. London 87 (1797) 159–196.

Halban, J.: Schwangerschaftsreaktionen der fötalen Organe und ihre puerperale Involution. Z. Geburtsh. Gynäkol. 53 (1904) 191–231.

Halban, J.: Die innere Sekretion von Ovarium und Plazenta und ihre Bedeutung für die Funktion der Milchdrüse. Arch. Gyn. 75 (1905) 353–441.

Hamblen, E. C.: Results of preoperative administration of extract of pregnancy urine: Study of ovaries and endometria in hyperplasia of endometrium following such administration. Endocrinology 19 (1935) 169.

Hamblen, E. C.: Clinical evaluation of ovarian responses to gonadotropic therapy. Endocrinology 24 (1939) 848.

Hamblen, E. C.: Endocrine therapy of functional ovarian failure. Am. J. Obstet. Gynec. 40 (1940) 615.

Hamblen, E. C., C. D. Davis: Treatment of hypo-ovarianism by the sequential and cyclic administration of equine and chorionic gonadotropins – so-called one-two cyclic gonadotropic therapy. Summary of five years' results. Am. J. Obst. & Gynec. 50 (1945) 137–146.

Hammerstein, J.: Hormonanalytische Untersuchungen zur Frage der endokrinen Korrelationen im biphasischen Menstruationszyklus der Frau. Arch. Gyn. 196 (1962) 504–540.

Hann, von F.: Über die Bedeutung der Hypophysenvorderlappenveränderungen bei Diabetes insipidus. Z. Pathol. 21 (1918) 337–365.

Harris, G. W., D. Jacobsohn: Functional grafts of the pituitary gland. Proc. R. Soc. Lond., Biol. 139 (1952) 263–276.

Hartree, A. S., J. B. Mills, R. A. S. Welc, M. Thomas: Fractionation of protein hormones from horse pituitary glands. J. Reprod. Fer. 17 (1968) 291–303.

Hayes, A., A. Johanson: Excretion of follicle-stimulating hormone (FSH) and luteinzing hormone (LH) in urine by pubertal girls. Pediat. Res. 6 (1972) 18–25.

Heinrichs, H. D., F. Eulefeld: Untersuchungen über die Extraktion von hypophysärem Gonadotropin aus Urin. Acta endocrinol. Suppl. 53 (1960) 5–48.

Heller, H.: History of neurohypophysial research. In Greep, R. O., E.B. Astwood: Handbook of Physiology. Endocrinology IV, part I (1974) 103–117.

Heller, C. G., Y. Clermont: Kinetics of the germinal epithelium in man. Rec. Progr. Horm. Res. 20 (1964) 545.

Hench, P. S., E. C. Kendall, Ch. Slocumb, H. F. Polley: The effect of a hormone of the adrenal cortex (17-hydroxy-11-dehydro-corticosteron, compund E) and if pituitary adrenocorticotropic hormone on rheumatoid arthritis. Proc. Mayo Cli. 24 (1949) 181–197 und 277–297.

Heynemann, Th.: Die Behandlung der juvenilen Blutungen. Zbl. Gynäk. 57 (1933) 2055.

Hertz, R., F. L. Hisaw: Effects of follicle-stimulating and luteinizing pituitary extracts on ovaries of infantile and juvenile rabbits. Am. J. Physiol. 108 (1934) 1–12.

Hill, M., A. S. Parkes: Proc. R. Soc. Lond. B 97 (1931) 291.

Hisaw, F. L., R. O. Greep, H. L. Fevold: Experimental ovulation of Macacus rhesus monkeys. Anat. Rec. Suppl. 61 (1935) 316–318.

Hobson, B.: The excretion of chorionic gonadotrophin by men with testicular tumours. Acta endocrinol. 49 (1965) 337–348.

Hofbauer, J.: Hypophysenextrakt als Wehenmittel. Zbl. Gyn. 35 (1911) 137–141.

Hofmann, K., H. Yajima, T. Y. Liu, N. Yanaihara: Studies on polypeptides. XXIV Synthesis and biological evaluatioan of a tricosapeptide possessing essentially the full biological activity of ACTH. J. Am. Chem. Soc. 84 (1962) 4475–4480.

Hofmann, K., H. Yajima, T. Y. Liu, N. Yanaihara, C. Yanaihara, J. L. Humes: Studies on polypeptides. XXV The adrenocorticotropic potency of an eicosapeptide amide corresponding to the N-terminal portion of the ACTH molecules; contribution to the relation between peptide chain lenght and biological activity. J. Am. Chem. Soc. 84 (1962) 4481–4486.

Hofmann, K.: Relation of the chemical structure and function of adrenocorticotropin and melanocyte-stimulating hormone. In Greep, R. O., E. B. Astwood (ed.): Handbook of Physiology. Section 7 Endocrinology. Am. Physiol. Soc., Washington (1974) 29–58.

Hoffmann, F.: Untersuchungen über die hormonale Regulation der Follikelreifung im Zyklus. Geburtsh. Frhkd. 21 (1961) 554–560.

Hoffmann, F.: Über die Wirkung des Progesterons auf das Follikelwachstum im Zyklus und seine Bedeutung für die hormonale Steuerung des Ovarialzyklus der Frau. Geburtsh. Frhkd. 22 (1962) 433–440.

Hofstätter, R.: Über Befunde bei hyperhypophysierten Tieren. Monatsschr. Geburtsh. Gynäkol. 49 (1919) 387–412.

Hohlweg, W., M. Dohrn: Beziehungen zwischen Hypophysenvorderlappen und Keimdrüsen. (Vortrag 2. Int. Congr. Sex Res., London 3.–9.8.1930). Wien. Arch. Inn. Med. 21 (1930) 337–350.

Hohlweg, W., K. Junkmann: Die hormonal-nervöse Regulierung der Funktion des Hypophysenvorderlappens. Klin. Wschr. 11 (1932) 321–323.

Hohlweg, W.: Veränderungen des Hypophysenvorderlappens und des Ovariums nach Behandlung mit großen Dosen von Follikelhormon. Klin. Wochenschr. 13 (1934) 92–95.

Hohlweg, W., A. Chamorro: Über die luteinisierende Wirkung des Follikelhormons durch Beeinflussung der endogenen Hypophysenvorderlappensekretion. Klin. Wochenschr. 16 (1937) 196–197.

Hornnes, P., D. Giroud, C. Howles, E. Loumaye: Recombinant human follicle-stimulating hormone treatment leads to normal follicle growth, estradiol secretion, and pregnancy in a WHO group II anovulatory woman. Fertil. Steril. 60 (1993) 724–726.

Horsley, V.: Functional nervous disorders due to loss of thyroid gland and pituitary body. Abstract of 3. Brown Lecture Lancet I (1886) 5.

Horsley, V.: Diseases of the pituitary gland. Br. Med. J. 1 (1906) 323.

Horsley, V.: On the technique of operations on the central nervous system. Br. Med. J. 2 (1906) 411–423.

Houssay, B. A., A. Biosotti, R. Sammartino: Modificationes fonctionelles de l'hypophyse après les lésion infundibulo tubériennes chez le capaud. C. R. Soc. Biol, Paris 120 (1935) 725–727.

Howell, W. H.: The physiological effects of extracts of the hypophysis cerebri and infundibular body. J. exptl. Med. 3 (1898) 245–258.

Hwang, P., H. Guyda, H. G. Friesen: A radioimmunoassay for human prolactin. Proc. Natl. Acad. Sci. 68 (1971) 1902–1906.

Igarashi, M., S. M. McCann: A new sensitive Bioassay for Follicle-stimulating hormone. Endocrinology 74 (1963) 440–445.

Illig, R., M: Zachmann, A. Prader: Menschliches Wachstumshormon. Klin. Wschr. 47 (1969) 117–123.

Insler, V., H. Melmed, I. Eichenbrenner, D.M. Serr, B. Lunenfeld: The cervical score – a simple semiquantitative method for monitoring of menstrual cycle. Int. J. Gynecol. Obstet. 10 (1972) 223–228.

Johansson, E. D. B., L. Wide: Periovulatory levels of plasma progesterone and luteinizing hormone in women. Acta endocr. 62 (1969) 82–88.

Johansson, E. D. B., L. Wide, C. Gemzell: Luteinizing hormone (LH) and progesterone in plasma and oestrogens in urine during 42 normal menstrual cycles. Acta endocr. 68 (1971) 502–512.

Johnsen, S. G.: The management of male hypogonadism. A clinical endocrinological synopsis. Acta endocrinol. Suppl. 66 (1962) 1.

Jones, G. S., Z. Aziz, G. Urbina: Clinical use of gonadotrophins in conditions of ovarian insufficiency of various etiologies. Fertil. Steril. 12 (1961) 217–235.

Jores, A.: Krankheiten der Hypophyse und des Hypophysenzwischenhirnsystem. In Linneweh, F. (Hrsg.): Stoffwechselkrankheiten. Handbuch der Inneren Medizin Bd. 7 / 1. Springer, Berlin, Göttingen, Heidelberg (1955).

Jungck, E. C., W. E. Brown: Human pituitary gonadotropin for clinical use: preparation and lack of antihormone formation. Fertil. Steril. 3 (1952) 224–229.

Junkmann, K., W. Schoeller: Über das thyreotrope Hormon des Hypophysenvorderlappen. Klin. Wchschr. 11 (1932) 1176–1177.

Jutisz, M., P. G. Squire: Occurrence of several active components in sheep pituitary interstitial cell-stimulating hormone, as evidenced by column electrophoresis. Bull. Soc. Chim. Biol. 40 (1958) 1875–1883.

Jutisz, M., P. G. Squire: Further evidence for the existence of several active components in sheep pituitary interstitial cell-stimulating hormone. Acta endocr. 37 (1961) 96–102.

Jutisz, M., C. Hermier, A. Colonge, R. Courrier: Purification et propriétés physico-chimiques et biologiques de l'hormone fulliculo-stimulante de Mouton. Annales d'Endocrinologie 26 (1965) 670–682.

Jutisz, M.: Jutisz Marian. In Bettendorf (Hrsg.): Zur Geschichte der Endokrinologie und Reproduktionsmedizin. Springer (1995) 274–284.

Kaiser, R., B. Mackert, W. Keyl: Die zeitliche Korrelation zwischen den Gonadotropin- und Östrogenmaxima und dem Basaltemperaturanstieg im Zyklus. Arch. Gyn. 199 (1964) 414–422.

Kallmann, F. J., W. A. Schönfeld: Psychiatric problems in the treatment of eunuchoidism. Am. J. Ment. Defic. 47 (1943) 203.

Kallmann, F. J., W. A. Schönfeld, S. E. Barrera: The genetic aspects of primary eunuchoidism. Am. J. Ment. Defic. 48 (1944) 386.

Kamm, O., T. B. Aldrich, I. W. Grote, L. W. Rowe, E. P. Bugbee: The active principles of the posterior lobes of the pituitary gland. J. Am. Chem. Soc. 50 (1928) 573–601.

Kaplan, N. M.: Successful pregnancy following hypophysectomy during the twelfth week of gestation. J. Clin. Endocr. Metabol. 21 (1961) 1139–1145.

Kaplan, S. L., M. M. Grumbach: The ontogenesis of human fetal hormones. II Luteinizing hormone (LH) and follicle stimulating hormone (FSH). Acta endocrinol. 81 (1976) 808–829.

Kaplan, S. L., M. M. Grumbach, M. L. Aubert: The ontogenesis of pituitary hormones and hypothalamic factors in the human fetus: maturation of central nervous system evulation of anterior pituitary function. Rec. Progr. Horm. Res. 32 (1976).

Kaplan, S. L., M. M. Grumbach, M. L. Aubert: α and β glycoprotein hormone subunits (hLH, hFSH, hCG) in the serum and pituitary of the human fetus. J. clin. Endocrinol. 42 (1976) 995–998.

Karg, H.: Ascorbinsäuredynamik im Ovar als Gonadotropinnachweis. Klin. Wochenschr. 35 (1957) 643–647.

Kaufmann, C.: Die Behandlung der Amenorrhö mit hohen Dosen der Ovarialhormone. Klin. Wschr. 12 (1933) 1557–1562.

Keller, P. J.: Die Bestimmung hypophysärer Gonadotropine im Urin. Gynaecologia 156 (1963) 380–389.

Keller, P. J., E. Rosemberg: Estimation of pituitary gonadotropins in human plasma. J. clin. Endocrinol. 25 (1965) 1050–1054.

Keller, P. J.: Studies on human pituitary gonadotrophins in human plasma. I. Normal values in men and women of all ages. II. Follicle stimulating and luteinizing hormone in male and female plasma. Acta endocrinol. 52 (1966) 341–347 und 348–354.

Keller, P. J.: Hypophysäre Gonadotropine. Untersuchungen über Physiologie, Pathologie und medikamentöse Beeinflussung der FSH- und LH-Sekretion bei der Frau. Fortschr. Geburtsh. Gynäkol. 44 (1971) 1–98.

Keene, J. L., M. M. Matzuk, T. Otani, B. C. J. M. Fauser, B. Galway, Hsueh: Expression of biologically active human follitropin in Chinese hamster ovary cells. J. Biol. Chem. 264 (1989) 4769–4775.

Kido, I.: Die menschliche Plazenta als Produktionsstätte des sogenannten Hypophysenvor- derlappenhormons (Experimentelle Untersuchungen). Zbl. Gyn. 61 (1937) 1551– 1555.

Knobil, E., R. O. Greep: Effects of growth hormone in normal and hypophysectomized rhesus monkeys. Federation Proc. 14 (1955) 86.

Knobil, E., R. O. Greep: The physiology of growth hormone with particular reference to its action in the rhesus monkey and the „species specifity" problem. Rec. Progr. Horm. Res. 15 (1959) 1–58.

Knobil, E., J. L. Kostyo, R. O. Greep: Production of ovulation in the hypophysectomized Rhesus Monkey. Endocrinology 65 (1959) 487–493.

Knobil, E., J. L. Kostyo, R. O. Greep: Action of gonadotrophins in hypophysectomized fe- male Rhesus monkeys. Fed. Proc. 17 (1959) 88.

Knobil, E.: On the regulation of the primate corpus luteum. Biol. Reprod. 8 (1973) 246.

Knobil, E.: On the control of gonadotrophin secretion in the rhesus monkey. Rec. Progr. Horm. Res. 30 (1974) 1.

Knobil, E.: The neuroendocrine control of the menstrual cycle. Rec. Progr. Horm. Res. 36 (1980) 53–88.

Knox, G. E., A. J. Dowd, S. A. Spiesel, R. Hong: Antihistamine blockade of the ovarian hy- perstimulation syndrome. II Possible role of antigen-antibody complexes in the patho- genesis of the syndrome. Fertil. Steril. 26 (1975) 418–420.

Knuth, U. A., W. Hönigl, M. Bals-Pratsch, G. Schleicher, E. Nieschlag: Treatment of severe oligospermia with human chorionic gonadotropin / human menopausal gonadotropin: a placebo-controlled, double blind trial. J. clin. endocrinol. Metab. 65 (1987) 1081– 1087.

Koenig, V. L., E. King: Extraction Studies of sheep pituitary gonadotropic and lactogenic hormones in alcoholic acetate buffers. Arch. biochem. 26 (1950) 219–229.

Konschegg, A., E. Schuster: Über die Beeinflussung der Diurese durch Hypophysenextrakte. Dt. Med. Wochschr. 41 (1915) 1091.

Kotz, H. L., W. Herrmann: A review of the endocrine induction of human ovulation. VI gonadotropins. Fertil. Steril. 12 (1961) 375–394.

Kracht, J., U. Hachmeister: Hormonbildungsstätten im Hypophysenvorderlappen des Menschen. Springer, Berlin, Heidelberg, New York, Dtsch. Ges. Endokrinol. (1969) 402–410.

Kraul, L.: Die Rückwirkung des Eierstocks auf den Hypophysenvorderlappen. Verh. Dt. Ges. Gynäk. 22 (1931) 452–455.

Kraul, L.: Die Beeinflussung der Hypophysenvorderlappenfunktion durch hormonale Substanzen und deren praktische Bedeutung. Arch. Gyn. 148 (1932) 65–75.

Kubik, C. J.: Luteal Phase Dysfunction following Ovulation Induction. Seminars in Repro- ductive Endocrinology 4 (1986) 293–300.

Kulin, H. E., A. B. Rifkind, G. T. Ross, W. D. Odell: Total gonadotropin activity in the uri- ne of prepubertal children. J. Clin. Endocr. 27 (1967) 1123–1128.

Kylin, E.: Ergebnisse von 24 Hypophysen-Transplantationen. Klin. Wochenschr. 15 (1936) 1756–1760.

Lastra, M. de la, C. Llados: Luteinzing hormone content of the pituitary gland in pregnant and non-pregnant women. J. Clin. Endocrinol. Metab. 44 (1977) 921–923.

League of Nations: Bull. Hlth. Org. L. o.N. 7 (1938) 894.

League of Nations: Bull. Hlth. Org. L. o.N. 8 (1939) 898.

Lee, T. H., A. B. Lerner, V. Buettner-Janusch: Adrenocorticotropic hormone and melanocyte-stimulating hormone from pituitary glands. Ciba Found. Colloqu. Endocrinol. 13 (1960) 251–265.

Lee, T. H., A. N. Lerner, V. Buettner-Janusch: On the structure of human corticotropin (adrenocorticotropic hormone). J. Biol. Chem. 236 (1961) 2970–2974.

Leung, P., B. H. Yuen, Y. S. Moon: Effect of prolactin in an experimental model of the ovarian hyperstimulation syndrome. Am. J. Obstet. 145 (1983) 847–849.

Levin, L., H. M. Tyndale: The quantitative assay of „Follicle stimulating" substances. Endocrinology 21 (1937) 619–623.

Levine, R. J., S. A. Metz: A classification of ectopic hormon-producing tumors. Ann. NY Acad. Sci. 230 (1974) 533–546.

Li, Ch. H., H. M. Evans, M. E. Simpson: Isolation of adrenocorticotropic hormone from sheep pituitaries. Science 96 (1942) 450.

Li, Ch. H., H. M. Evans, M. E. Simpson: Adrenocorticotrophic hormone. J. biol. Chem. 149 (1943) 413–424.

Li, C. H., H. M. Evans: The isolation of pituitary growth hormone. Science 99 (1944) 183–184.

Li, C. H., H. M. Evans, M. E. Simpson: Isolation and properties of anterior hypophyseal growth hormone. J. Biol. Chem. 159 (1945) 353–366.

Li, C. H.: The chemistry of gonadotropic hormones. Vitamins and Hormones I (1949) 223.

Li, Ch. H., H. Papkoff: Preparation and properties of growth hormone from human and monkey pituitary glands. Science 124 (1956) 1293–1294.

Li, Ch. H.: Properties of and structural investigations on growth hormones isolated from bovine, monkey and human pituitary glands. Fed. Proc. 16 (1957) 775–783.

Li, Ch. H.: Growth Hormone from monkey and human pituitaries. Cancer 10 (1957) 698–703.

Li, M. C., R. Hertz, D. M. Bergenstral: Therapy of choriocarcinoma and related trophoblastic tumors with folic acid and purine antagonist. N. Engl. J. Med. 259 (1958) 66–70.

Li, C. H.: Purification of follicle-stimulating hormone from human pituitary glands. Proc. Soc. exp. Biol., NY 98 (1958) 839–841.

Li, Ch. H.: Studies on human pituitary growth and gonadotropic hormone. Endocrinology 13 (1960) 46–64.

Li, Ch. H., P. G. Squire, U. Gröschel: Purification and properties of human follicle-stimulating and interstitial cell-stimulating hormone. Arch. Biochem. Biophys. 86 (1960) 110–116.

Li, Ch. H.: The biochemistry of prolactin. In Kon, S. K., A. T. Cowie (ed.): Milk: The mammary gland and its secretion. Acad. Press, New York, chapt. 5 (1961) 205–228.

Li, Ch. II., J. S. Dixon, D. Chung: Adrcnocorticotropins. XXI Thc amino acid sequence of bovine adrenocorticotropin. Biochem. Biophys. Acta 46 (1961) 324–344.

Li, Ch. H., B. Starman: Molecular weight of sheep pituitary interstitial cell-stimulating hormone. Nature 202 (1964) 291–292.

Li, Ch. H.: Lipotropin a new active peptide from pituitary glands. Nature, Lond. 201 (1964) 924.

Li, Ch. H., J. S. Dixon, T. B. Lo, Y. A. Pankov, K. D. Schmidt: Amino acid sequence of ovine lactogenic hormone. Nature 224 (1969) 695–696.

Li, Ch. H., J. S. Dixon: Human pituitary growth hormone. XXXII. The primary structure of the hormone. Arch. Biochem. Biophys. 46 (1971) 233–236.

Li, Ch. H.: Recent knowledge of the chemistry of lactogenic hormones. In Wolstenholme, G. E. W., J. Knight (ed.): Lactogenic Hormones. Ciba Foundation, London (1972) 7–26.

Li, Ch. H., D. Chung: Primary structure of human β-lipotropin. Nature 260 (1976) 623–625.

Licht, P., H. Papkoff: Gonadotrophic activities of the subunits of ovine FH and LH in the lizard Anolis caroliensis. Gen. & comp. Endocr. 16 (1971) 586.

Licht, P.: Action of mammalian pituitary gonadotropins (FSH and LH) in Reptiles I. Male Snakes 273–281. II. Turtles 282–289 (1972).

Licht, P., H. Papkoff, S. W. Farmer, C. H. Muller, H. W. Tsui, D. Crews: Evolution of gonadotropin structure and function. Rec. Progr. Horm. Res. 33 (1977) 169–248.

Lichtenberg, V., V. Pahnke: Measurement of biologically active LH / HCG in vitro Testosterone Production assay (TPA) and problems when applied to serum. Acta endocrinol. Suppl. 202, 82 (1976) 54–57.

Lichtenberg, V.: Biologische Bestimmung von Lutropin (LH) in Serum und Hypophyse mit Hilfe isolierter Maus-Leydigzellen. Dissertation Hamburg, Fachbereich Biologie (1980).

Lichtenberg, V., H. C. Weise, D. Graesslin, G. Bettendorf: Polymorphism of human pituitary lutropin (LH), Effect of the seven isohormones on mouse Leydig cell functions. FEBS letters 169 (1984) 21–24.

Lichtwitz, L.: Drei Fälle von Simmondscher Krankheit (hypophysäre Kachexie). Klin. Wochenschr. 1 (1922) 1873–1879.

Liddle, G. W., W. E. Nicholson, D. P. Island et al.: Clinical and laboratory studies of ectopic humoral syndromes. Rec. Prog. Horm. Res. 25 (1969) 283–314.

Little, B., O. W. Smith, A. G. Jessiman, H. A. Selenkow, W. Vant Hoff, J. M. Eglin, F. D. Moore: Hypophysectomy during pregnancy in a patient with cancer of the breast: Case report with hormone studies. J. Clin. Endocr. Metabol. 18 (1958) 425–443.

Louwerens, B. (ed.): Menschliche Gonadotropine, neue Erfahrungen aus Laboratorium und Klinik. Rundtischgespräch im Tel-Hashomer Government Hospital 28. Mai 1968. Acta endocrinol. 64, Suppl. 148 (1970).

Lunenfeld, B., A. Menzi, B. Volet: Clinical effects of human postmenopausal gonadotrophin. 1. Int. Congr. Endocrinology Copenhagen, Advance Abstracts of short Communications, Periodica Copenhagen 587 (1960).

Lunenfeld, B., E. Rabau, G. Rumney, G. Winkelsberg: The responsivness of the human ovary to gonadotrophin. III. Weltkongr. Int. Fed. Gynäk. Geburtsh. Wien Bd. II 220 (1961).

Lunenfeld, B., S. Sulimovici, E. Rabau, A. Eshkol: L'induction de L'ovulation dans les amenorrhées hypophysaires par un traiment combiné de gonadotrophines urinaires menopausiques et de gonadotrophines chorioniques. C. R. Soc. Franc. Gynecol. 32 (1962) 346–351.

Lunenfeld, B.: Treatment of anovulation by human gonadotrophins. J. Int. Fed. Gyn. Obstet. 1 (1963) 153–167.

Lunenfeld, B., V. Insler, M. Glezerman: Diagnosis and treatment of functional infertility. Grosse Verlag, Berlin (1978).

Lunenfeld, B., D. Olchovsky, D. Tadir, M. Glezerman: Treatment of male infertility with human gonadotrophins; selection of cases, management and results. Andrologia 11 (1979) 331–336.

Lunenfeld, B., D. M. Serr, S. Mashiach, G. Oelsner, J. Blankstein, J. Dor, Y. Frenkel, Z. Ben-Raphael, D. Tikotzky, M. Snyder: Therapy with Gonadotropins: Where are we today? Analysis of 2890 Menotopin Treatment Cycles in 914 patients. In Insler, V., G. Bettendorf, K. H. Geissler (ed.): Advances in Diagnosis and Treatment of Infertility. Elsevier / North Holland (1981) 27–32.

Lups, T.: Anat. Anz. Jena 67 (1929) 161.

Luukainen, T., H. Adlerkreutz, R. Vihko, G. Bettendorf: Plasma and urinary steroids in hypophysectomized women during treatment with gonadotropins. In Bettendorf, G., V. Insler (ed.): Clinical application of human gonadotropins. Thieme, Stuttgart (1970) 134–150.

MacLeod, J. A., A. Pazianos, B. Ray: Restoration of human spermatogenesis by menopausal gonadotrophins. Lancet 1 (1964) 1197.

MacLeod, J. A., A. Pazianos, B. Ray: The restoration of human spermatogenesis and of the reproductive tract with urinary gonadotrophins following hypophysectomy. Fertil. Steril. 17 (1966) 7–10.

Maddock, W. O.: Antihormone formation complicating pituitary gonadotropin therapy in infertile men I. Properties of the antihormones. J. clin. Endocr. 9 (1949) 213.

Magnus, R., E. A. Schäfer: The action of pituitary extracts upon the kidney. J. Physiol. London 27 (1901) 9–10.

Mahnert, A.: Hypophysenvorderlappen und Ovarium. Tierexperimentelle Untersuchungen über das Bestehen von wechselseitiger Beziehung zwischen dem Ovarium und dem Hypophysenvorderlappen. Zbl. Gyn. 52 (1928) 1754–1758.

Mancini, R. E.: Effect of different types of gonadotrophins on the induction and restoration of spermatogenesis in the human. Acta Europ. Fertil. 1 (1969) 401–405.

Marie, P.: Sur deux cas d'acromégalie. Hypertrophie singulière non congénitale des extremités supérieures, inférieures et céphaliques. Rev. Méd. 6 (1886) 297–333.

Marie, P., J. D. Souza-Leite: Essays on Acromegaly. London, New Sydenham Society (1891).

Martial, J. A., R. A. Hallewell, J. D. Baxter, H. M. Goodman: Human growth hormone: complementary DNA cloning and expression in bacteri. Science 205 (1979) 602–607.

Matikainen, T., R. de Leeuw, B. Mannaerts, I. Huhtaniemi: Circulating bioactive and immunoreactive recombinant human follicle-stimulating hormone (Org. 32489) after administration to gonadotropin-deficient subjects. Fertil. Steril. 61 (1994) 62–69.

Matsuo, H., Y. Baba, R. G. M. Nair, A. Arimura, A. Schally: Structure of porcine LH and FSH releasing hormone. 1 The proposed amino acid sequence. Biochem. Biophys. Res. Comm. 43 (1971) 1334–1339.

Mazer, C., E. Ravetz: The effect of combined administration of chorionic gonadotropin and the pituitary synergist on the human ovary. Am. J. Obstet. Gynec. 41 (1941) 474.

McArthur, J. W.: The identification of pituitary interstitial cell stimulating hormone in human urine. Endocrinology 50 (1952) 304–310.

McArthur, J. W., R. B. Pennell, H. N. Antoniades, F. M. Ingersoll, H. Ulfelder: The distribution of pituitary gonadotropin in fractions of human plasma. Proc. 39th meeting of the Endocrine Society. Abstract 15, (1957) 100.

McArthur, J. W., F. M. Ingersoll, J. Worcester: Urinary excretion of interstitial-cell stimulating hormone by normal males and females of various ages. J. clin. Endocrinol. 18 (1958) 460–469.

McArthur, J. W., J. Worcester, F. M. Ingersoll: The urinary excretion of interstitial-cell and follicle-stimulating hormone activity during the normal menstrual cycle. J. Clin. Endocrinol. Metab. 18 (1958) 1186–1201.

McArthur, J. W., H. N. Antoniades, L. H. Larson, R. B. Pennell, F. M. Ingersoll, H. Ulfelder: Follicle-stimulating hormone and luteinizing hormone content of pooled human plasma and of subfractions prepared by Cohn method 6 and 9. J. Clin. Endocrinol. Metab. 24 (1964) 425–431.

McArthur, J. W.: An animal model for the induction of ovulation by means of gonadotropin treatment. In Rosemberg, E. (ed.): Gonadotropins in female infertility. Excerpta Med. Congr. Ser. 266 (1973) 77–83.

McCann, S. M., S. Taleisnik, H. M. Friedman: LH releasing activity in hypothalamic extracts. Proc. Soc. Exp. Biol. Med. 104 (1960) 432–434.

McCann, S. M.: A hypothalamic luteinizing releasing hormone-releasing factor. Am. J. Physiol. 202 (1962) 395–400.

Meier, A. H., R. MacGregor: Temporal Organization in Avian Reproduction. Am. Zoologist 12 (1972) 257–271.

Meigs, J. V., J. W. Cass: Fibroma of the ovary with ascites and hydrothorax. Am. J. Obstet. Gynecol. 33 (1937) 240–267.

Meites, J.: Prolactin. In Endocrinology, People and Ideas. Am. Physiol. Soc. Bethesda, Ma. (1988) 117–147.

Meldrum, D. R.: Low dose follicle stimulating hormone therapy for polycystic ovarian disease (editorial). Fertil. Steril. 55 (1991) 1039–1040.

Merz, W. E., V. Hilgenfeldt, M. Dörner, R. Brossmer: Biological, immunological and physical investigations on human chorionic gonadotropin. Hoppe Seyler's Z. Physiol. Chem. 355 (1974) 1035.

Midgley, A. R., R. B. Jaffe: Regulation of human gonadotropins: X. Episodic fluctuation of LH during the menstrual cycle. J. Clin. Endocr. 33 (1971) 962–969.

Moore, C. R., D. Price: The question of sex hormone antagonism. Proc. Soc. Exp. Biol. Med. 28 (1930) 38–40.

Moore, C. R., D. Price: Gonad hormone functions and the reciprocal influence between gonads and hypophysis, with its bearing on sex hormone antagonism. Am. J. Anat. 50 (1932) 13–71.

Morgan, F. J., R. E. Canfield: Nature of the subunits of human chorionic gonadotropin. Endocrinology 88 (1971) 1045–1053.

Morgan, F. J., R. E. Canfield: The primary structure of the HCG-α subunit. In IVth Int. Congr. Endocrinology, Excerpta Med. Congr. Ser. (1973).

Morgan, F. J., R. E. Canfield: Human chorionic gonadotropin – A proposal for the amino acid sequence. Moll. Cell. Biochem. 2 (1973) 97.

Morgan, F. J., R. E. Canfield, J. L. Vaitukaitis, G.T. Ross: Properties of the subunits of human chorionic gonadotropin. Endocrinology 94 (1977) 1601.

Morris, C. J. O. R.: Chemistry of the Gonadotrophins. Brit. Med. J. 11 (1955) 101–104.

Morris, C. J. O. R.: The Chemistry of Gonadotrophins. In Parkes, A. S. (ed.): Marshalls Physiology of Reproduction. Little Brown, Boston (1966) 379–411.

Moses, M., H. Bogowsky, E. Anteby, B. Lunenfeld, E. Rabau, D. Serr, A. David, M. Salomy: Thromboembolic phenomena after ovarian stimulation with human gonadotropins. Lancet 2 (1965) 1213–1215.

Muller, P.: Vor- und Nachteile der hochkonzentrierten Choriongonadotropin-Präparate. Gynaecologia 152 (1961) 341–347.

Murata, M., K. Adachi: Über die künstliche Erzeugung des Corpus luteum durch Injektion der Plazentarsubstanz aus frühen Schwangerschaftsmonaten. Z. Geburtsh. Gynäk. 92 (1927) 45.

Nelson, D. H., J. W. Meakin, J. W. Thorn: ACTH producing pituitary tumours following adrenalectomy for Cushing's Syndrome. Ann. Int. Med. 52 (1960) 560–567.

Neuwirth, R. S., R. N. Turksoy, Vande Wiele: Acute Meig's syndrome secondary to ovarian stimulation with human menopausal gonadotropins. Am. J. Obstet. Gynec. 91 (1965) 977.

Niepce, B.: Traite du goitre et du cretinisme. Paris (1851).

Niswender, G. D., A. R. Midgley, S. E. Monroe, L. E. Reichert: Radioimmunoassay for rat luteinizing hormone with antiovine LH serum and ovine LH-131 I. Proc. Soc. Exp. Biol. Med. 128 (1968) 807–811.

Niswender, G. D., C. L. Chen, A. R. Midgley, J. Meites: Radioimmunoassay for rat prolactin. Proc. Soc. Exp. Biol. Med. 130 (1969) 793–797.

Nikovitch-Winer, M., J. W. Everett: Functional restitution of pituitary grafts re-transplanted from kidney to median eminence. Endocrinology 63 (1958) 916–930.

Nitschke-Dabelstein, S., G. Strum, B. J. Hacklelör, E. Daume, R. Buchholz: Welchen Stellenwert besitzt die endokrinologische Überwachung in der Gonadotropinstimulierung anovulatorischer Patientinnen – ein Vergleich zwischen endokrinologischen und ultrasonographischen Parametern. Geburtsh. u. Frauenheilk. 40 (1980) 702–712.

Noble, G. K., K. F. Kumpf, V. N. Billings: The induction of brooding behavior in fish. Anat. Record. Suppl. 67 (1936) 50.

Novak, E., G. B. Hurd: Use of pituitary luteinizing substance in treatment of functional uterine bleeding. Am. J. Obstet. Gynec. 22 (1931) 501–512.

Novales, R. R.: Actions of melanocyte-stimulating hormone. In Greep, R. O., E. B. Astwood (ed.): Handbook of Physiology, Section 7 Endocrinology. Am. Physiol. Soc. Washington (1974) 347–366.

Nydick, M., R. J. Berry, W. D. Odell: Molecular weight of human chorionic gonadotropin as estimated by means of radiation inactivation of biologic activity. J. Clin. Endocr. 24 (1964) 1049–1054.

Odell, W. D.: Melanocyte-stimulating Hormones, Lipotropins, the Endorphins, and enkephalin. In DeGroot, L. J.: Endocrinology. Grune & Stratton, NY, San Francisco, London (1979) 169–173.

Oliver, G., E. A. Schäfer: On the physiological actions of extracts of the pituitary body and certain other glandular organs. J. Physiol. London 18 (1895) 277–279.

Olson, J. L., R. W. Rebar, J. R. Schreiber, J. L. Vaitukaitis: Shortened luteal phase after ovulation induction with human menopausal gonadotropin and human chorionic gonadotropin. Fertil. Steril. 39 (1983) 284–290.

Omenn, G.: Pathobiology of ectopic hormone production by neoplasms in man. Pathobiol. Annu. 3 (1973) 177–216.

Oppenheim, Herrmann: Diskussion in Arch. Psychiat. Nervenkr. 34 (1901) 303–304.

Opri, F., G. Post, H. Kirchner, J. Hammerstein: Bestimmung des HCG im Serum und in Zystenpunktaten bei verschiedenen Formen der Mastopathie. Geburtsh. Frauenheilk. 39 (1979) 690–693.

Østergaard, E.: Antigonadotrophic substances under treatment with gonadotrophic hormones. E. Munksgaard, Copenhagen (1942) 1–184.

Ott, I., J. C. Scott: The action of infundibulum upon the mammary secretion. Proc. Soc. Exp. Biol. Med. 8 (1910) 48.

Ovadia, J., J. W. McArthur, O. W. Smith, J. Bashir-Fahrahmand: An individualized technique for induction ovulation in the bonnet monkey, Macaca radiata. Reprod. Fertil. 27 (1971) 13–23.

Page, R. B.: The Anatomy of the hypothalamo-hypophyseal complex. In Knobil, E., J. Neill et al.: The Physiology of Reproduction. Raven Press, New York (1988) 1161–1233.

Palmer, A.: Chorionic Gonadotropin. Its Place in the treatment of infertility. Fertil. Steril. 8 (1957) 220.

Papkoff, H., Ch. H. Li, W. K. Liu: The isolation and characterization of growth hormone from porcine pituitaries. Arch. Biochem. Biophys. 96 (1962) 216–225.

Papkoff, H., T. S. A. Samy: Isolation and partial characterization of polypeptide chains of ovine interstitial cell stimulating hormone. Biochim. Biophys. Acta 147 (1967) 175–177.

Papkoff, H., D. Gospodarowicz, Ch. H. Li: Purification and properties of ovine follicle-stimulating hormone. Arch. Biochem. Biophys. 120 (1967) 434–439.

Papkoff, H., N. R. Sairam, C. H. Li: Amino sequences of the subunits of ovine interstitial-stimulating hormone. J. Am. chem. Soc. 93 (1971) 1531.

Papkoff, H.: Structure of follicle stimulating hormone. In IVth Int. Congr. Endocrinology, Excerpta Med. Congr. Ser. (1973).

Papkoff, H., M. R. Sairam, S. W. Farmer, C. H. Li: Studies on the structure and function of interstitial-stimulating hormone. Rec. Progr. Horm. Res. 29 (1973) 563–590.

Papkoff, H., R. J. Ryan, D. N. Ward: The Gonadotropic Hormones, LH (ICSH) and FSH. In Greep, R. O., M. A. Koblinsky (ed.): Frontiers in Reproduction and Fertility Control. The MIT Press, Cambridge, Mass and London, England (1977) 1–10.

Papkoff, H.: Remembrance: Glycoprotein hormones were always composed of subunits – we just had to find out the hard way. Endocrinology 129 (1991) 579–581.

Parkes, A. S.: The rise of reproductive endocrinology 1926–1940. The Sir Henry Dale Lecture for 1965. J. Endocrinol. 34 (1965) XX–XXXII.

Parlow, A. F.: A rapid bioassay method for LH and factors stimulating LH secretion. Fed. Proc. 17 (1958) 402.

Parlow, A., L. Reichert: Biological assay of Luteinizing hormone (LH, ICSH) by the ovarian hyperemia method of Ellis. An Evaluation. Endocrinology 72 (1963) 944–961.

Parlow, A., L. E. Reichert: Species differences in follicle-stimulating hormone as revealed by the slope in the Steelman-Pohley assay. Endocrinology 73 (1963) 740–743.

Paulesco, N. C.: L'Hypophyse du Cerveau. J. Physiol. Pathol. Gen. 9 (1907) 441–456.

Paulesco, N. C.: L'Hypophyse du Cerveau. Vigot Frères, Eds. Paris (1908).

Paulsen, C. A., D. H. Espeland, E. L. Michals: Effects of hCG hMG, hLH, and hGH administration on testicular function. In Rosemberg, E., C. A. Paulsen (eds.): The Human Testis. Plenum Press, New York (1970) 547.

Pearse, A. G.: Observation on the localisation, nature and chemical constitution of some components of the anterior hypophysis. J. Pathol. Bacteriol. 64 (1952) 791.

Pearse, A. G., S. van Noorden: The functional cytology of the human adenohypophysis. Can. Med. Ass. J. 88 (1963) 462.

Pfeiffer, C.: Sexual differences of the hypophysis and their determination by the gonads. Am. J. Anat. 58 (1936) 195–222.

Philipp, E.: Die Bildungsstätten des Hypophysenvorderlappenhormons in der Gravidität. Zentrbl. Gynäkol. 54 (1930) 1858–1866.

Philipp, E.: Hypophysenvorderlappen und Plazenta. Zbl. Gynäkol. 54 (1930) 450–453.

Philipp, E.: Hypophysenvorderlappen oder Plazenta? Zbl. Gynäkol. 57 (1933) 2237–2240.

Phillips, L. L., W. Glanstone, R. vande Wiele: Studies of the coagulation and fibrinolytic systems in hyperstimulation syndrome after administration of human gonadotropins. J. Reprod. Med. 14 (1975) 138–140.

Pierce, J. C., L. K. Wynston, M. E. Cartsen: Studies on the purification of thyrotropin. Biochim. Biophs. Acta 28 (1958) 434–435.

Pierce, J. G., T. H. Liao, S. M. Howard, B. Shome, J. S. Cornell: Studies on the structure of thyrotrophin: its relationship to luteinizing hormone. Recent. Progr. Horm. Res. 27 (1971) 165–212.

Pietsch, K.: Aufbau und Entwicklung der Pars tuberalis des menschlichen Hirnanhangs in ihren Beziehungen zu den übrigen Hypophysenteilen. Z. mikrosk. anat. Forsch. 22 (1930) 227–257.

Polishuk, W. Z., J. G. Schenker: Ovarian overstimulation syndrome. Fertil. Steril. 20 (1969) 443–450.

Popa, G. T., U. Fielding: A portal circulation from the pituitary to the hypothalamic region. J. Anat. Lond. 65 (1930) 88–91.

Porchet, H.C., J. Y. le Cotonnec, E. Loumaye: Clinical pharmacology of recombinant human follicle-stimulating hormone. III. Pharmacokinetic-pharmacodynamic modeling after repeated subcutaneous administration. Fertil. Steril. 61 (1994) 687–695.

Prader, A.: Zur Behandlung des hypophysären Zwergwuchses. In Klein, E. (ed.): Wachstumshormon und Wachstumsstörungen, das Cushing-Syndrom. Springer, Berlin, Göttingen, Heidelberg (1965) 68–80.

Pride, S. M., B. H. Yuen, Y. S. Moon: Clinical, endocrinological, and intraovarian prostaglandin F responses to H-1 receptor blockade in the ovarian hyperstimulation syndrome. Studies in the rabbit model. Am. J. Obstet. Gynecol. 148 (1984) 670–674.

Purves, H. D.: Cytology of the Adenohypophysis. In Harris, G. W., B. T. Donovan: The Pituitary Gland. Vol. I Butterworths, London (1966) 147–232.

Rabau, E., A.David, D. M. Serr, S. Mashiach, B. Lunenfeld: Human menopausal gonadotropin for anovulation and sterility. Am. J. Obstet. Gynecol. 92 (1967) 92–96.

Raben, M. S.: Preparation of growth hormone from pituitaries of man and monkey. Science 125 (1957) 883.

Raben, M. S.: Treatment of a pituitary dwarf with human growth hormone. J. Clin. Endocr. 18 (1958) 901.

Rathke, M. H.: Über die Entstehung der Glandula pituitaria. Archiv für Anatomie, Physiol. Wiss. Med., Müllers Archiv, (1838) 482–485.

Rauscher, H.: Untersuchungen über den luteotropen Effekt hoher Choriongonadotropindosen bei der Frau. Geburtsh. Frauenheilk. 15 (1955) 265.

Reichert, L. E.: Preparation of purified bovine luteinizing hormone. Endocrinology 71 (1962) 729–733.

Reichert, L. E.: Preparation of ovine follicle-stimulating hormone having a high degree of biological purity. Endocrinology 73 (1963) 224–229.

Reichert, L. E., N. S. Jiang: Comparative gelfiltration and density gradient centrifugation studies on heterologous pituitary luteinizing hormone. Endocrinology 77 (1965) 78–86.

Reichert, L. E., N. S. Jiang: Studies on bovine pituitary follicle-stimulating hormone. Endocrinology 77 (1965) 124–127.

Reid, R. L., N. Ling, S. S. C. Yen: Melanocyte stimulating hormone induces gonadotropin release. J. clin. Endocrinol. 52 (1981) 159–161.

Reisfeld, R. A., R. Hertz: Purification of chorionic gonadotropin from the urine of patients with trophoblastic tumors. Biochim. Biophys. Acta 43 (1960) 540–543.

Reinboth, R.: Hormonal Control of the Teleost Ovary. Am. Zoologist 12 (1972) 307–324.

Report of the Council on Pharmacy and Chemistry: Chorionic gonadotropin. JAMA 114 (1940) 2306–2307.

Reye, E.: Das klinische Bild der Simmondschen Krankheit (hypophysäre Kachexie) in ihrem Anfangsstadium und ihre Behandlung. MMW 73 (1926) 902–906.

Reye, E.: Die ersten klinischen Symptome bei Schwund des Hypophysenvorderlappens und ihre erfolgreiche Behandlung. Dtsch. Med. Wochenschr. 54 (1928) 696–697.

Reye, E.: Klinik und Therapie der Simmondschen Krankheit und verwandter Zustände. Zentralbl. Med. 41 (1931) 946.

Rice, B. F., R. Ponthier, W. Sternberg: Luteinizing hormone and growth hormone activity of the human fetal pituitary. J. clin. endocr. metabol. 28 (1968) 1071–1072.

Riddle, O., P. F. Braucher: Studies on the physiology of reproduction in birds. XXX. Control. of the special secretion of the crop gland in pigeons by an anterior pituitary hormone. Am. J. Physiol. 97 (1931) 617–625.

Riddle, O., R. W. Bates, S. W. Dykshorn: A new hormone of the anterior pituitary. Proc. Soc. Exptl. Biol. Med. 29 (1932) 1211–1215.

Riddle, O., R. W. Bates, S. W. Dykshorn: The preparation, identification and assay of prolactin – a hormone of the anterior pituitary. Am. J. Physiol. 105 (1933) 191–216.

Riddle, O., R. W. Bates, E. L. Lahr: Prolactin induces broodiness in fowl. Am. J. Physiol. 111 (1935) 352–360.

Riddle, O., E. L. Lahr, R. W. Bates: Maternal behavior induced in virgin rats by prolactin. Proc. Soc. Exptl. Biol. Med. 32 (1935) 730–734.

Riddle, O.: Comments. In Smith, R. W. jr., O.H. Gaebler, C. N. H. Long (ed.): The Hypophyseal growth hormone. Nature and Actions. MacGraw-Hill, New York (1955) 495–496.

Rifkind, A. B., H. E. Kulin, P. L. Rayford, C. M. Cargille, G. T. Ross: 24-hour urinary luteinizing hormone (LH) and follicle-stimulating hormone (FSH) excretion in normal children. J. Clin. Endocr. 31 (1970) 517–525.

Riisfeldt, O.: Methods and results in 117 cases of amenorrhoea treated with gonadotropic hormones. Acta Obstet. Gynec. Scand. 29 (1949) 255–290.

Rocca, D., A. Albert: Daily urinary excretion of follicle-stimulating hormone during the menstrual cycle. Mayo Clin. Proc. 42 (1967) 536–546.

Romeis, B.: Die Hypophyse. In Mollendorf J. (ed.): Handbuch der mikroskopischen Anatomie des Menschen. Springer, Berlin Vol.6 (1940).

Ron, E., B. Lunenfeld, J. Menczer, T. Blumstein, L. Katz, G. Oelsner, D. Serr: Cancer incidence in a cohort of infertile women. Am. J. Epidemiol. 125 (1987) 780–790.

Rosemberg, E., J. Coleman, M. Demany, C. R. Garcia: Clinical effects of human urinary postmenopausal gonadotropin. J. Clin. Endocr. 23 (1963) 181.

Rosemberg, E., J. Coleman, N. Gibree, W. MacGillivray: Clinical effect of gonadotropins of human origin. Fertil. Steril. 13 (1962) 220–236.

Rosemberg, E., J. Engel: Comparative activities of two preparations from the urine of postmenopausal women. J. clin. Endocr. 21 (1961) 1063.

Rosemberg, E., P. J. Keller: Studies on the urinary excretion of follicle-stimulating and luteinizing hormone activity during the menstrual cycle. J. Clin. Endocrin. Metabol. 25 (1965) 1262–1274.

Ross, G. T.: Clinical relevance of research on the structure of human chorionic gonadotropin. Am. J. Obstet. Gynecol. 129 (1977) 795–808.

Ryan, R. J.: The luteinizing content of human pituitaries. I. Variations with sex and age. J. Clin. Endocrinol. Metab. 22 (1962) 300–303.

Rydberg, E., V. Madsen: The treatment of functional sterility with gonadotropic hormones. Acta Obstet Gynec. Scand. 28 (1949) 386–402.

Rydberg, E., E. Østergaard: The effect of gonadotropic hormone treatment in cases of amenorrhoea. Acta Obstet. Gynec. Scand. 19 (1939) 222–246.

Rydberg, E., Pedersen-Bjergaard: Effect of serum gonadotropin and chorionic gonadotropin on the human ovary. J. Am. med. Ass. 121 (1943) 1117–1122.

Saffran, M., A. V. Schally, B. G.Benfry: Stimulation of the release of corticotropin from the adenohypophysis by a neurohypophysial factor. Endocrinology 57 (1955) 439–444.

Sairam, M. R., A. F. Papkoff, C. H. Li: Human pituitary interstitial cell stimulating hormone: Primary structure of the alpha subunit. Biochem. Biophys. Res. Commun. 48 (1973) 530–537.

San Juan, A. M.: Falta total de los nervios olfactorios con anosmia en un individuo en quien ecista una atrofia congenita de los testiculos y miembro viril. Siglomedico, Madrid (1856) 211.

Santomé, J. A., J. M: Dellacha, A. C. Paladini, C. E. M. Wolfenstein, C. Pena, E. Porkus, S. T. Daurat, M. J. Biscoglio, Z. M. M. De Sesé, A. V. F. Sanguesa: The amino acid sequence of bovine growth hormone. FEBS Letters 16 (1971) 198–200.

Saxena, B. B., P. Rathnam: Purification and properties of human pituitary FSH. In Rosemberg E.: Gonadotropins. Geron-X Los-Altos, Calif. (1968) 3–12.

Sayers, G., M. A. Sayers, A. White, C. N. H. Long: Effect of pituitary adrenotropic hormone on cholesterol content of rat adrenal glands. Proc. Soc. Exptl. Biol. Med. 52 (1943) 200–202.

Sayers, G., A. White, C. N. H. Long: Preparation and properties of pituitary adrenotropic hormone. J. biol. Chem. 149 (1943) 413–424 und 425–436.

Sayers, G., M. A. Sayers, H. L. Lewis, C. N. H. Lomg: Effects of adrenotropic hormone on ascorbic acid and cholesterol content of the adrenal. Proc. Soc. Eptl. Biol. Med. 55 (1944) 238–239.

Sayers, G., M. A. Sayers, L. A. Woodbury: The assay of adrenocorticotrophic hormone by the adrenal ascorbic acid-depletion method. Endocrinology 42 (1944) 379–393.

Scanes, C. G., S. Dobson, B. K. Follett, J. M. Dodd: Gonadotrophic activity in the pituitary gland of the dogfisch (Scyliorhinus Canicula). J. Endocr. 54 (1972) 343–344.

Schäfer, E. A., S. Vincent: On the action of extract of pituitary injected intravenously. J. Physiol. London 24 (1899) XIX–XXI.

Schäfer, E. A., S. Vincent: The physiological effects of extracts of the pituitary body. J. Physiol. London 25 (1899) 87–97.

Schäfer, E. A., P. T. Herring: The action of pituitary extracts upon the kidney. Phil. Trans. Roy Soc. London 199 (1908) 1–29.

Schäfer, E. A., K. Mackenzie: The action of animal extracts of milk secretion. Proc. Roy Soc. London Ser. B 84 (1911) 16–22.

Schäfer, E. A.: On the effect of pituitary and corpus luteum extracts on the mammary gland in the human. Quart. J. eypl. Physiol. 4 (1913) 17–19.

Scharrer, E. A., B. Scharrer: Hormones produced by neurosecretory cells. Rec. Progr. Horm. Res. 101 (1954) 183–240.

Scharrer, E. A.: Principles of neuroendocrine integration. Res. Publ. Assoc. Nerv. Ment. Dis. 43 (1966) 1–35.

Schipperges, H.: Die Entwicklung der Hirnchirurgie. Ciba Z. Bd. 7 (1955) 2470–2498.

Schloffer, H.: Erfolgreiche Operation eines Hypophysentumors auf nasalem Wege. Wien. klin. Wochenschr. 20 (1907) 621–624.

Schockaert, J. A., H. Siebke: Gehalt des menschlichen Hypophysenvorderlappens an gonadotropen Hormonen. Zbl. Gyn. 47 (1932) 2774–2782.

Schönberg, D., J. R. Bierich: Über das Wachstumshormon. Arch. Kinderheilkunde 173 (1966) 226–237.

Schönemann, A.: Hypophysis und Thyreoidea. Arch. path. Anat. 129 (1892) 310–336.

Schüller, A.: Röntgen-Diagnostik der Erkrankungen des Kopfes. Alfred Hölder, Wien und Leipzig (1912).

Schwanzel-Fukula, M., D. Bick, D. W. Pfaff: Luteinizing hormone-releasing hormone (LHRH) – expressing cells do not migrate normally in an inherited hypogonadal (Kallmann) syndrome. Mol. Brain. Res. 6 (1989) 311–326.

Schwyzer, R., P. Sieber: Total synthesis of adrenocorticotrophic hormone. Nature 199 (1963) 172–174.

Sciarra, N., U. Leone: Urinary excretion of luteinizing hormone in boys and adult men. J. Endocr. 46 (1970) 229–236.

Scott, A. P., P. J. Lowrey: Adrenocorticotrophic and melanocyte stimulating peptides in the human pituitary body. Biochem. J. 139 (1974) 593–597.

Seeburg, P. H., J. Shine, J. A. Martial, A. Ullrich, H. M. Goodman, Baxter: Nucleotide sequence of human gene coding for a polypeptide hormone. Trans. Assoc. Am. Physicians 90 (1977) 109–116.

Seeburg, P. H., J. Shine, J. A. Martial, R. D. Ivarie, J. A. Morris, A. Ullrich, J. D. Baxter, H. M. Goodman: Synthesis of growth hormone by bacteria. Nature 176 (1978) 795–798.

Seibel, M. M., M. Kamrava, C. McArdle, M. L. Taymor: Treatment of polycystic ovarian disease with chronic low-dose follicle stimulating hormone: biochemical changes, and ultrasound correlation. Int. J. Fertil. 29 (1984) 39–43.

Sheehan, H. L.: Post partum necrosis of the anterior pituitary. J. Pathol. Bacteriol. 45 (1937) 189–214.

Sheehan, H. L.: Simmonds Disease due to post partum necrosis of the anterior pituitary. Q. J. Med. 8 (1939) 277–309.

Shome, B., A. F. Parlow: The primary structure of the hormone-specific β subunit of human pituitary luteinizing hormone (hLH). J. Clin. Endocrinol. Metab. 36 (1973) 618–621.

Shome, B., A. F. Parlow: Human pituitary prolactin (hPRL): the entire linear amino acid sequence. J. Clin. Endocrinol. Metab. 45 (1977) 1112–1115.

Siebke, H.: Behandlung juveniler Blutungen mit Hypophysenvorderlappenhormon. Mschr. Geburtsh. Gynäk. 95 (1933) 298.

Siegmund, H.: Über den Einfluß des Hypophysenvorderlappens auf den Ablauf der Sexualfunktion. Zbl. Gyn. 52 (1928) 1189–1196.

Simmer, H. H.: Die Erschließung der endokrinen Funktion der Plazenta. I. Halbans Hypothese von 1903 / II. Halbans klassische Arbeit von 1905. Endokrinologische Informationen 6 (1984) 249–266 und 1 (1985) 25–39.

Simmonds, M.: Über Hypophysenschwund mit tödlichem Ausgang. Dtsch. Med. Wochenschr. 40 (1914) 322–323.

Simmonds, M.: Atrophie des Hypophysenvorderlappens und hypophysäre Kachexie. Dtsch. Med. Wochenschr. 44 (1918) 852–853.

Simpson, M. E., G. van Wagenen, F. Carter: Hormone content of anterior pituitary of monkey (Macaca mulatta) with special reference to gonadotrophins. Proc. Soc. Exp. Biol. Med. 91 (1956) 6–11.

Simpson, M. E., G. Wagenen: Experimental induction of ovulation in the rhesus monkey. Endocrinology 61 (1958) 316–318.

Simpson, M. E., G. Wagenen: Induction of ovulation with human urinary gonadotrophin in the monkey. Fertil. Steril. 13 (1962) 140–152.

Smith, P. E.: Experimental ablation of the hypopyhsis in the frog embryo. Science, N. Y. 44 (1916) 280–282.

Smith, P. E.: The effect of hypophysectomy in the early embryo upon growth and development of the frog. Anat. Record. 11 (1916) 57–64.

Smith, P. E., I. P. Smith: The Repair and Activation of the Thyroid in the Hypophysectomized Tadpole by the parenteral Administration of fresh anterior Lobe of the Bovine Hypophysis. J. M. Research 43 (1922) 267–283.

Smith, P. E., I. P. Smith: The function of the lobes of the hypophysis and indicated by replacement therapy with different portions of the Ox-gland. Endocrinology 7 (1923) 579–591.

Smith, P. E.: Hastening development of female genital system by daily homoplastic pituitary transplants. Proc. Soc. exp. Biol. Med. 24 (1926) 131–132.

Smith, P. E.: Ablation and transplantation of the hypophyses in the rat. Anat. Record. 32 (1926) 221.

Smith, P. E.: The disabilities caused by hypophysectomy and their repair, The tuberal (hypothalamic) syndrome in the rat. J. Am. med. Assoc. 88 (1927) 158–161.

Smith, P. E., E. T. Engle: Experimental evidence regarding the role of the anterior pituitary in the development and regulation of the genital system. Am. J. Anat. 40 (1927) 159–217.

Smith, P. E.: Hypophysectomy and replacement therapy in the rat. Am. J. Anat. 45 (1930) 205–274.

Smith, P. E., E.T. Engle: Gonad-stimulating hormones from the pituitary and from human urine. J. Pediat. 5 (1934) 163–176.

Smith, P. E., E. T. Engle, H. H. Tyndale: Gametokinetic action of extract of folliclestimulating urine. Proc. Soc. Exp. Biol. Med. 31 (1934) 745–746.

Smith, P. E., S. L. Leonhard: Responses of reproductive system of hypophysectomized and normal rats to injection of pregnancy-urine extracts. I. the male. Anat. Rec. 58 (1934) 145–170.

Smith, P. E.: Continuation of pregnancy in Rhesus Monkeys (Macaca mulatta) following hypophysectomy. Endocrinology 55 (1954) 655–664.

Snyder, P. J., F. H. Sterling: Hypersecretion of LH and FSH by a pituitary adenoma. JCE & M 42 (1976) 544–550.

Soemmering, Th. von: Dissertatio de basi encephali et originibus nervorum cranio egredientium libri quinque. Göttingen (1778).

Squire, P. G., C. H. Li: Purification and properties of an interstitial cell-stimulating hormone from sheep pituitaries. Science 127 (1958) 32.

Squire, P. G., Ch. H. Li, R. N. Andersen: Purification and characterization of human pituitary intestitial cell-stimulating hormone. Biochemistry 1 (1962) 412–418.

Staemmler, H.J.: Die gestörte Regelung der Ovarialfunktion. Springer, Berlin, Göttingen, Heidelberg (1964).

Steelman, S. L., F. M. Pohley: Assay of the follicle stimulating hormone based on the augmentation with human chorionic gonadotropin. Endocrinology 53 (1953) 604–616.

Steelman, S. L.: Chromatography of follicle-stimulating hormone on hydroxyl apatite. Biochim. Biophys. Acta 27 (1958) 405–406.

Steelman, S. L., A. Segaloff, R. Andersen: Purification of human pituitary follicle stimulating and luteinizing hormones. Proc. Soc. Exp. Biol. Med. 101 (1959) 452–454.

Steelman, S. L., A. Segaloff: Recent studies on the purification of pituitary gonadotropins. Rec. Progr. Horm. Res. 15 (1959) 115–125.

Sterneck, M., D. Graesslin, V. Lichtenberg, G. Bettendorf: The complete polymorphism of human pituitary FSH and comparison of the isohormone pattern between males and females. Acta endocrinol. 114, Suppl. 283 (1987) 41.

Stewart, H. L.: Hormone Secretion by human placenta grown in the eyes of rabbits. Am. J. Obstet. Gynecol. 61 (1951) 990–1000.

Stewart, J., C. H. Li: On the use of -tropin or - trophin in connection with anterior pituitary hormones. Science 137 (1962) 336–337 und 138, 728–730.

Storring, P. L., H. Dixon, D. R. Bangham: The first international standard for human urinary FSH and for human urinary LH (ICSH), for bioassay. Acta endocrinol. 83 (1976) 700–710.

Storring, P. L., R. E. Gaines-Das, D. R. Bangham: International Reference Preparation of human chorionic gonadotrophins for immunoassay: potency estimates in various bioassay and protein binding assay systems; and international reference preparation of the α and β subunits of human chorionic gonadotrophin for immunoassay. J. Endocr. 84 (1980) 295–310.

Storring, P. L., R. E. G. Das: The second International Standard for Human Pituitary LH: its collaborative study by bioassays and immunoassays. J. Endocrinol. 138 (1993) 345–359.

Stricker, P., F. Grüter: Action du lobe anterieur de l'hypophyse sur la montee laiteuse. Compt. Rend. Soc. Biol. 99 (1928) 1978–1980.

Strott, C. A., T. Yoshimi, G. T. Ross, M. B. Lipsett: Ovarian physiology: relationship between plasma LH and steroidogenesis by the follicle and corpus luteum; effect of HCG. J. Clin. Endocr. 29 (1969) 1157–1167.

Swyer, G. I. M., V. Little, D. Lawrence, J. Collins: Gonadotrophin stimulation test of ovarian function. Brit. Med. J. 1 (1968) 319–352.

Tandler, J., S. Groß: Über den Einfluß der Kastration auf den Organismus. Wien. Klin. Wochenschr. 20 (1907) 1596–1597.

Tandler, J., S. Groß: Untersuchungen an Skopzen. Wien. Klin. Wochenschr. 21 (1908) 277–288.

Taymor, M. L.: Timing of ovulation by LH assay. Fertil. Steril. 10 (1959) 212–226.

Taymor, M. L.: Excretion of follicle stimulating hormone and interstitial-cell stimulating hormone in different phases of the normal menstrual cycle. J. clin. Endocrinol. 21 (1961) 976–984.

Taymor, M. L., S. H. Sturgis: Induction of ovulation with human postmenopausal gonadotropin. II Possible causes of overstimulation. Fertil. Steril. 17 (1966) 736–741.

Taymor, M. L., S. H. Sturgis, D. P. Goldstein, B. Lieberman: Induction of ovulation with human postmenopausal gonadotropin. III Effect of varying dosage schedules on estrogen and pregnanediol excretion levels. Fertil. Steril. 18 (1967) 181–190.

Taymor, M. L.: Gonadotropin Therapy, Possible Causes and Prevention of Overstimulation. Am. J. Med. Ass. 203 (1968) 362–364.

Taymor, M. L., B. Lieberman, T. H. Rizkallah: FSH excretion during the normal menstrual cycle. Fertil. Steril. 20 (1969) 267–274.

Thompson, C. R., L. M. Hansen: Pergonal (menotropins): A summary of clinical experience in the induction of ovulation and pregnancy. Fertil. Steril. 21 (1970) 844–853.

Townsend, S. L., J. B. Brown, J. W. Johnstone, F. D. Adey, J. H. Evans, H. P. Taft: Induction of ovulation. J. Obstet. gynecol. Br. Commonw. 73 (1966) 529.

Tscherne, E.: Die Behandlung der weiblichen Sterilität mit gonadotropen Hormonen. Wien. klin. Wschr. 69 (1957) 890.

Turner, R. A., J. G. Pierce, V. du Vigneaud: The purification and amino acid content of vasopressin preparations. J. biol. Chem. 191 (1951) 21–28.

Utiger, R. D., M. L. Parker, W. H. Daughaday: Studies on human growth hormone. I. A radioimmunoassay for human growth hormone. J. Clin. Investig. 41 (1962) 254–261.

Vaitukaitis, J. L.: Immunologic and physical characterization of human chorionic gonadotropin secreted by tumors. JCE & M 37 (1973) 505–514.

Vaitukaitis, J. L., E. R. Ebersole: Evidence for altered synthesis of human chorionic gonadotropin in gestational trophoblastic tumors. JCE & M 42 (1976) 1048–1055.

Van Damme, M. P., D. M. Robertson, R. Marana, E. M. Ritzén, E. Diczfalusy: A sensitive and specific in vitro bioassay method for the measurement of follicle-stimulating hormone activity. Acta endocrinol. 91 (1979) 224–237.

Van Hell, H., B. C. Goverde, A. H. W. M. Schuurs, E. de Jager, R. Matthijsen, J. D. H. Homan: Purification, characterization and immunochemical properties of human chorionic gonadotropin. Nature 212 (1966) 261–262.

Velden, von den R.: Beiträge zur Wirkung von Hypophysenextrakten. Berlin. Klin. Wochschr. 50 (1913) 1969.

Velden, von den R.: Die Nierenwirkung von Hypophysenextrakten beim Menschen. Berlin. Klin. Wochschr. 50 (1913) 2083–2086.

Venturoli, S., R. Fabbri, R. Paradisi, O. Magrini, E. Porcu, L. F. Orsini, C. Flamigni: Induction of ovulation with human urinary follicle-stimulating hormone: Endocrine pattern and ultrasound monitoring. Europ. J. Obstet. Gynec. Reprod. Biol. 16 (1983) 135–145.

Venturoli, S., R. Fabbri, R. Paradisi, P. Mimmi, F. Franceschetti, G. Bolelli, C. Flamigni: Induction of ovulation with „pure" humanurinary FSH in patients with chronic anovulation and polycystic ovaries. In Flamigni, C., J. R. Givens (eds.): The Gonadotropins. Academic Press, London, New York (1982) 439–450.

Venturoli, S., R. Paradisi, R. Fabbri, O. Magrini, E. Porcu, C. Flamigni: Comparison between human urinary FSH and HMG treatment in polycystic ovary. Obstet. Gynecol. 63 (1984) 6–11.

Vigneaud, du V., C. Ressler, J. M. Swan et al.: The synthesis of an ocatapeptide amide with the hormone activity of oxytocin. J. Am. Chem. Soc. 75 (1953) 4879–4880.

Vigneaud, du V.: Hormones of the posterior pituitary gland: oxytocin and vasopressin. Harvey Lectures, Ser. 50 (1954–1955) 1–26.

Vigneaud, du V., M. F. Bartlett, A. Johl: The synthesis of lysine-vasopressin. J. Am. Chem. Soc. 79 (1957) 5572–5575.

Vigneaud, du V., D. T. Gish, P. G. Katsoyannis, G. P. Hess: Synthesis of the pressor-antidiuretic hormone, arginine-vasopressin. J. Am. Chem. Soc. 8 (1958) 3355.

Vöge, A.: Neue Wege in der Behandlung der glandulär-cystischen Hyperplasie. Arch. Gynäk. 174 (1943) 1–45.

Vogt, M.: Nervous influences in endocrine activity. In Meites, J. et al. (ed.): Pioneers in Neuroendocrinology. Vol. 1 (1975) 314–321.

Vozza, F.: Über die Herkunft der sogenannten Hypophysenvorderlappenhormone in der Schwangerschaft. Z. Geburtsh. Gynäk. 102 (1932) 468–472.

Wagenen, G. van, M. E. Simpson: Gonadotrophic hormone excretion of the pregnant monkey. Proc. Soc. Exp. Biol. Med. 90 (1955) 346–348.

Wagenen, G. van, M.E. Simpson: Experimentally induced ovulation in the rhesus monkey (Macacca mulatta). Rev. Suisse Zool. 64 (1957) 809–819.

Wahlén, T.: Studies of metropathia haemorrhagica cystica. Acta Obstet. Gynec. Scand 29, Suppl. 6 (1950) 1–202.

Walborg, E. F., D. N. Ward: The carbohydrate components of ovine luteinizing hormone. Biochim. Biophys. Acta 78 (1963) 304–312.

Ward, D. N., M. Fujino, M. Showalterm, N. Ray: Comparative studies of luteinizing hormone from beef, pork and sheep pituiteries I. purification and physical properties. Gen & compar. Endocr. 8, 44–53. II. The C-terminal amino acids 8 (1967) 289–296.

Ward, D. N., L. E. Reichert, W. K. Liu, H. S. Nalin, J. Hesia, W. M. Lamkin, N. S. Jones: Chemical studies of luteinizing hormone from human and ovine pituitaries. Rec. Progr. Horm. Res. 29 (1973) 533.

Weintraub, B. D., S. W. Rosen: Competitive radioassays and „specific" tumor markers. Metabolism 22 (1973) 1119–1127.

Weise, H. C., D. Graesslin, V. Lichtenberg, G. Rinne: Polymorphism of human pituitary lutropin (LH). Isolation and partial characterisation of seven isohormones. FEBS letters 159 (1983) 93–96.

Wepfer, J. J.: Observationes anatomicae, ex cadaveribus eorum, quos sustulit apoplexia. Schaffhausii, J. C. Suteri (1658).

Wepfer, J. J.: Observationes anatomicae ex Cadaveribus. Amsterdam (1681).

Westman, A.: Untersuchungen über den Einfluß der Hormone des Hypophysenvorderlappen auf die Funktion des Corpus luteum. Zbl. Gynäk. 56 (1932) 450–456.

Westman, A.: Untersuchungen über die Wirkung des gonadotropen Hypophysenvorderlappenhormons „Antex" (Leo) auf die Ovarien der Frau. Acta Obstet Gynec. Scand. 17 (1937) 492–515.

Westman, A.: Die gonadotropen Hormone und ihre therapeutische Anwendung. Geburtsh. u. Frauenheilk. 2 (1940) 595–609.

Westman, A., D. Jacobsohn: Endokrinologische Untersuchungen an Ratten mit durchtrenntem Hypophysenstiel. I. Hypophysenveränderungen nach Kastration und nach Oestrinbehandlung. Acta Obst. Gynecol. Scand. 18 (1938) 99–108.

Wezenbeek, P. van, J. Draaijer, F. van Meel, W. Olijve: Recombinant FSH I. Construction, selection and characterization of a cell line. In Crommelin, D. J. A., H. Schellekens (ed.): From Clone to clinic, developments in biotherapy. Vol. 1 Dordrecht, Germany, Kluwer (1990) 245–251.

Wide, L., C. A. Gemzell: An immunological pregnancy test. Acta Endocrinol. 35 (1960) 261–267.

Wide, L., P. Roos, C.A. Gemzell: Immunological determination of human pituitary luteinizing hormone (LH). Acta Endocrinol. 37 (1961) 445–449.

Wide, L.: An immunological measure for the assay of chorionic gonadotropin. Acta Endocrinol. Suppl. 70 (1962) 1–111.

Wide, L., C. Gemzell: Immunological determination of pituitary luteinizing hormone in the urine of fertile and postmenopausal women and adult men. Acta endocr. 39 (1962) 539.

Wide, L.: Radioimmunoassays employing immunosorbents. In Diczfalusy, E. (ed.): Immunoassay of gonadotrophins. Acta endocrinol. Suppl. 142 (1969) 207–221.

Wide, L.: Follicle-stimulating hormones in anterior pituitary glands from children and adult differ in relation to sex and age. J. Endocrinol. 123 (1989) 519–529.

Wiesner, B. P., F. A. E. Crew: On the separation of kyogenic hormone from human placenta. Proc. roy. Soc. Edinb. 50 (1930) 79.

Wilhelmi, A. E., J. B. Fishman, J. A. Russel: A new preparation of crystalline anterior pituitary growth hormone. J. Biol. Chem. 176 (1948) 735–745.

Wirz, P.: Hypophysenvorderlappen und Amenorrhö. Z. Geburtsh. 104 (1933) 293–322.

Wislocki, G. B., L. S. King: The permeability of the hypophysis and the hypothalamus to vital dyes, with a study of the hypophysial vascular supply. Am. J. Anat. 58 (1936) 421–472.

World Health Organization Expert Committee on Biological Standardization. Wld. Hlth. Org. techn. Rep. Ser. 222 (1961) 9.

World Health Organization Expert Committee on Biological Standardization. Wld. Hlth. Org. techn. Rep. Ser. 293 (1964) 11.

World Health Organization: WHO Scientific Group on Agents Stimulating Gonadal Function. Technical Report Ser. No. 514 (1973).

World Health Organization: Expert Committee on biological standardization. 26th report, Technical Report Ser. TRS 565 (1975).

Würterle, A., W. Schmidt: Hormonuntersuchungen im mensuellen Zyklus. Zbl. Gyn. 81 (1959) 1389–1390.

Yen, S. S. C., C. C. Tsai, F. Naftolin, G. Vandenberg, L. Ajabor: Pulsatile patterns of gonadotropin release in subjects with and without ovarian function. J. Endocrinol. Metab. 34 (1972) 671–675.

Yazaki, K., C. Yazaki, K. Wakabayashi, M. Igarashi: Isoelectric heterogeneity of human chorionic gonadotropin: presence of choriocarcinoma specific components. Am. J. Obstet. Gynecol. 138 (1980) 189–194.

Yoshimoto, Y., A. R. Wolfsen, F. Hirose, W. D. Odell: Human chorionic gonadotropin-like material: presence in normal human tissues. Am J. Obstet. Gynecol. 134 (1979) 729–733.

Zander, R.: Über funktionelle und genetische Beziehungen der Nebennieren zu anderen Organen, speziell zum Großhirn. Beitr. Patol. Anat. 7 (1890) 439–534.

Zondek, B.: Über die Funktion des Ovariums. Zschr. Geb. Gynäk. 90 (1926) 372–380.

Zondek, B., S. Aschheim: Das Hormon des Hypophysenvorderlappens. 1. Testobjekt zum Nachweis des Hormons. Klin. Wschr. 6 (1927) 248–252.

Zondek, B., S. Aschheim: Das Hormon des Hypophysenvorderlappens. Darstellung, chemische Eigenschaften, biologische Wirkungen. Klin. Wochenschr. 7 (1928) 831–835.

Zondek, B.: Über die Hormone des Hypophysenvorderlappens. Klin. Wochenschr. 9 (1930) 245–248.

Zondek, B.: Zur gonadotropen Stimulationstherapie. Prolan, Synprolan, Prosylan. Acta Obstet. Gynec. Scand. 15 (1936) 1–11.

Zondek, B., F. G. Sulman: The antigonadotrophic factor with consideration of the antihormone problem. Williams & Wilkins Co., Baltimore (1942) 1–185.

Zondek, B.: Professor Bernhard Zondek, an interview. J. Reprod. Fert. 12 (1966) 3–19.

Zuckerman, S.: The secretions of the brain; relation of hypothalamus to pituitary gland. Lancet 1 (1954) 739–795.